# Manual Medicine
Therapy

# Manual Medicine
## Therapy

Werner Schneider, Jiří Dvořák
Václav Dvořák and Thomas Tritschler

Translated and edited by
Wolfgang G. Gilliar and Philip E. Greenman
Foreword by Mark Mumenthaler
327 Illustrations

1988
Georg Thieme Verlag Stuttgart · New York
Thieme Medical Publishers, Inc., New York

Werner Schneider, M.D.
FMH Physical Medicine, Rheumatology
Hauptstr. 39
CH-8280 Kreuzlingen
Switzerland

Jiří Dvořák, M.D.
Dept. of Neurology
Wilhelm Schulthess Hospital
Neumünsterallee 3
CH-8008 Zürich
Switzerland

Václav Dvořák, M.D.
General Practice
Bahnhofstr. 10
CH-7402 Bonaduz
Switzerland

Thomas Tritschler, P.T.
Director, School for Physical Therapy
Kantonsspital
CH-8208 Schaffhausen
Switzerland

Translators:
Wolfgang G. Gilliar, D.O.
National Rehabilitation Hospital
102 Irving Street, N.W.
Washington, D.C. 20010, USA

Philip E. Greenman, D.O.
Professor
College of Osteopathic Medicine
Michigan State University
East Lansing, 48823, USA

*Library of Congress Cataloging-in-Publication Data*

Manuelle Medizin--Therapie. English.
  Manual medicine--therapy.
  Translation of: Manuelle Medizin--Therapie.
  Includes bibliographies and index.
  1. Manipulation (Therapeutics)
I. Schneider, W. (Werner), 1941 –
II. Gilliar, Wolfgang G. III. Greenman, Ph. E.,
1928 – . IV. Title. [DNLM: 1. Manipulation,
Orthopedic. 2. Physical Medicine.
WB 460 M2937]
RM724.M3613   1988   615.8'22   88–2241

This Book is an authorized translation from the German edition published and copyrighted 1986 by Georg Thieme Verlag, Stuttgart, West Germany.
Title of the German edition: Manuelle Medizin – Therapie

**Important Note:** Medicine is an ever-changing science. Research and clinical experience are continually broadening our knowledge, in particular our knowledge of proper treatment and drug therapy. Insofar as this book mentions any dosage or application, readers may rest assured that the authors, editors and publishers have made every effort to ensure that such references are strictly in accordance with the state of knowledge at the time of production of the book. Nevertheless, every user is requested to carefully examine the manufacturers' leaflets accompanying each drug to check on his own responsibility whether the dosage schedules recommended therein or the contraindications stated by the manufacturers differ from the statements made in the present book. Such examination is particularly important with drugs which are either rarely used or have been newly released on the market.

© 1988 Georg Thieme Verlag, Rüdigerstrasse 14,
D-7000 Stuttgart 30, West Germany
Printed in West Germany
Typesetting (System 5, Linotron 202) by Druckhaus Dörr,
D-7140 Ludwigsburg
Printed by K. Grammlich, Pliezhausen

ISBN 3-13-713901-5 (GTV)
ISBN 0-86577-266-5 (TMP)

# Foreword

The anatomic and pathophysiologic fundamentals of manual medicine have already been presented by these authors in a previous book "Manual Medicine – Diagnostics". This book on therapy in manual medicine is the continuation of the other work, and much like the diagnostic text, it convincingly presents a justifiable, understandable, conclusive, quantifiable and reproducible treatment modality.

First, the basic concepts and mechanisms of manual therapy, as well as the indications for it, are presented in a self-critical way. This is followed by a presentation of the therapeutic techniques for each of the spinal segments and also for other joints.

The clarity of the overall book structure, the lucid organization of the individual sections and the logical, systematic way in which the authors approach the therapeutic procedures is exemplary. This book once again shows how an empirically discovered method of therapy can become a science through systematic analysis. Only then can it be passed on, and only then does it become understandable and therefore teachable. The authors have applied their intelligence to endow the desire to heal with the concrete form of manual medicine.

"The urge to heal can only be the motive and the driving force behind our actions; the direction of these actions, the decision of where and how, is solely a matter of understanding."
(E. Bleuler: Das autistisch-undisziplinierte Denken in der Medizin und seine Überwindung, 1921) (title translated: The Autistic – Undisciplined Thinking In Medicine and How To Overcome It.)

May this excellent book serve as an advisor for many doctors, chiropractors and physical therapists in their therapeutic work, and set an example to many an author. But let us hope that the reader will find the patience and humility to consistently and self-critically practice the methods he has theoretically learnt and understood, to ever refine and improve the therapeutic techniques of manual medicine.

Berne                                        Mark Mumenthaler

V

# Preface

A reviewer of one of our earlier works warned us that, as practitioners of manual medicine, we should not be quite so explicit in expressing the fear of coming into contact with traditional medicine and their representatives. It has always been our intent to present the basic principles of manual medicine as they pertain to diagnosis and therapy in a manner and style understandable by and familiar to physicians in the various other specialties. The documentation of our work is intended to break down the resentments that exist between manual medicine, traditional medicine and chiropractic, the roots of which can be found, in Switzerland at least, in the opinions on chiropractic by the Zurich and Berne Faculties (1936, 1937, respectively).

In the eyes of the observer, manual medicine has developed at an amazing rate during the last twenty years. A large number of doctors, physical therapists and chiropractors receive better and more comprehensive training today. The great interest shown by practicing colleagues is not just due to the quality of the training one receives nowadays in the field of manual medicine but also the therapeutic results that can be achieved utilizing this treatment modality. Manual Medicine has found its applications in general practice, physical medicine and rehabilitation, rheumatology, orthopedics and neurology.

Together with the previous volume MANUAL MEDICINE – DIAGNOSTICS, this text intends to present the current concepts of manual medicine practice.

We would like to emphasize, however, that manual therapy, although a significant part in the overall treatment of functional and degenerative disorders affecting the spine, joints and muscles, should be seen in the context of a larger framework of treatment. Each practitioner will also make use of his or her own, and quite often specialized training, so as to present to the patient a form of treatment that is the combination of all the practitioners skills including those of psychology and manual medicine. The guideline of good medical practice then becomes "Primum nil nocere" – above all, do no harm.

At this point we would like to express our thanks to our teachers and friends who introduced us to the field of manual medicine and its closely related specialties such as physcial medicine and rehabilitation, rheumatology, neurology, orthopedics. All those who supported this undertaking we thank sincerely. Our special thanks go to H. Cavizel, M.D., who introduced us to manual medicine. We further want to thank our teachers K. Lewit, M.D., and Prof. V. Janda, M.D., for their ideas and introduction to the field.

Furthermore, and again, we want to extend our thanks to Ph. Greenman, D.O., and W. Gilliar, D.O., for their diligence and constructive criticism during the preparation of the English edition.

We want to thank Ms. J. Reichert for doing the secretarial work and Ms. I. Hannweber and Ms. B. Schneider for their help during the revisions and corrections of the manuscript. Rezila Medical Furniture Limited and Fanco & Co. Ltd. loaned us the treatment tables and supported us with the photographic work.

Our grateful thanks again go to Georg Thieme Verlag, especially Mr. A. Menge, for the assistance concerning the graphic design of the book.

Kreuzlingen and Berne, Switzerland    W. Schneider
January, 1988    J. Dvořák
   V. Dvořák
   T. Tritschler

# Contents

# Contents

# Contents

# 1 Manual Therapy: Concepts and Mechanisms of Action

Manual medicine has been known to supplement and contribute to other medical specialities, especially such fields as conservative orthopedics, physical medicine, neurologic and rheumatologic rehabilitation. Within the field of manual medicine itself, there have been identified certain treatment procedures that, because of their known potential risks, require special attention and thus, should be performed only by licensed practitioners, such as allopathic and osteopathic physicians and chiropractors. In particular, the techniques associated with certain risks include the classic manipulation procedures, also known as "thrust" techniques or now called the mobilization with impulse techniques. It is the task and duty of the licensed practitioner to recognize both the absolute and relative contraindications to manipulative therapy. The physical therapist is neither trained nor authorized to discern the contraindications, because an in-depth clinical assessment alone may often not be suffcient. The physician only can judge if and what further diagnostic workup is in order and follow up accordingly, i.e., radiographs, laboratory tests, etc. On the other hand, the nonthrust techniques, also known in more general terms as the soft tissue techniques and most recently called the mobilization techniques without impulse, are those that have proved rather useful to the field of physical therapy. Both the mobilization techniques with and without impulse require an exact anatomic, biomechanic, and neurophysiologic understanding of the locomotor system.

Manipulative therapy in Europe has experienced significant growth and development within the past decades. This may be partially attributable to the interest demonstrated by a small group of physicians who have taken an interest in this treatment modality. Also the fact that osteopathic physicians in the United States were granted the same practicing privileges as their allopathic colleagues has probably contributed to this development.

Manual medicine, as practiced in Europe in the 1950s and 1960s, resorted primarily to techniques that had been presented by John Menell and the chiropractors trained in the United States. These classic manipulation techniques, that is, the mobilization techniques with impulse, had often been referred to by both the public and the sceptical physicians as "bone cracking." More and more frequently, however, patients with back pain turned with great hope to the chiropractors as well as to those physicians practicing manual medicine, a trend that continued especially when the exclusive use of myotonolytic and analgetic treatment procedures had not fulfilled the original expectations.

Even though the efficacy of manipulative therapy has not been proven in double-blind studies, there exist indications that this form of therapy can shorten the painful exacerbations of functional locomotor disturbances, which in turn significantly diminishes work absenteeism. In Switzerland, for instance, 1.5 million work days are lost annually due to back pain alone. Back pain or degenerative changes affecting the vertebral column are the second most frequent cause of partial or full disability in Switzerland.

In the 1970s, and in particular the 1980s, the field of manual medicine began to analyze its successes and failures, searching for neurophysiologic explanations that could illustrate the effect of manipulative treatment. Furthermore, terms such as "subluxation" and "somatic lesion" were no longer acceptable in the scientific language, requiring necessary and specific changes. As more and more manipulations were performed, it became apparent that the patient's symptoms could be improved immediately; however, in many cases the frequency of symptomatic recurrences seemed not to be influenced. It is believed that significant stimulation of the mechanoreceptors, as it is thought to occur with manipulation, causes presynaptic inhibition of the nociceptive afferent impulses at the level of the posterior horn of the spinal cord. In four scientific studies, encephalins are believed to be involved in this inhibitory process. At this time, however, one is unable to answer the question if, for example in the cervical spine, the classic manipulation procedures in actuality do set free a jammed meniscoid or if specific rotation movements displace the nucleus pulposus unloading the apophyseal joints and nerve roots. It is also not known to what extent intradiscal pressure will be increased with manipulation.

Therefore, the following questions need to be raised:
- How often should manipulation to the apophyseal be performed?
- Is it possible to prevent relapses and if so, what are the specific procedures?

Even though a final answer to these questions cannot be presented at this time, the establishment of muscular balance appears to play a great role in the prevention of recurrences. Important in manual treatment are such aspects as the stretching of the shortened tonic muscles, the strengthening of the weak phasic muscle groups, as well as specific instructions for a home exercise program.

Some of the classic thrust techniques, i.e., mobilization with impulse, needed modification, as with time adverse reactions and even significant complications have become known. The good contact between the European schools and the osteopathic physcians in the United States helped both introduce and integrate the mobilizing techniques without impulse into the treatment program in Europe. These techniques intend to introduce stretch to the noncontractile structures, such as ligaments and joint capsules. It is conceivable that these mobilization techniques may displace the nucleus pulposus as well.

More recently, there has heen the trend to conceptualize the locomotor system as the neuromusculoskeletal system, a concept that is also reflected in the field of manual therapy. Neuromuscular therapy (NMT), for instance, utilizing the reflexogenic mechanisms of the postisometric relaxation of the agonistic muscles and the reciprocal inhibition of the antoagonistic muscles, has found a permanent place within modern manual medicine. Also, of benefit is the fact that the patient actively particpates in his treatment.

Due to the complexity of the abnormal movements and motor patterns associated with the spinal or the extremity joints, it is necessary that very specific and different treatment procedures be applied in each case, utilizing the entire biomechanic and functional anatomic knowledge.

## 1.1 Introduction, Definitions

- *Angular Motion:* During both active and passive movement, the rolling-gliding motion is the physiologic motion in a joint or spinal segment. The joint anatomy, along with the arrangement of the ligaments and muscles, determines the direction and extent of this roll-glide motion (Fig. **1**). Using a three-dimensional coordinate system, one can construct three axes about which rotation can take place, designated as x, y, z.

    Flexion, extension = rotation about the x-axis
    Inclination, reclination (C0–C2) = rotation about the x-axis (specific terms used to designate flexion or extension in C0–C1–C2)
    Rotation = rotation about the y-axis
    Side-bending = rotation about the z-axis
    Abduction, adduction
    Elevation, depression

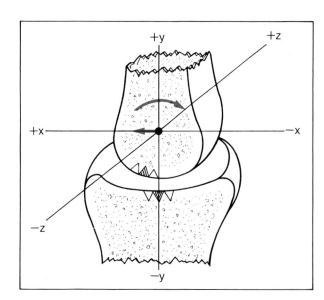

Figure **1** Angular motion:
+x   gliding
+⌀z rotation (about the z-axis)

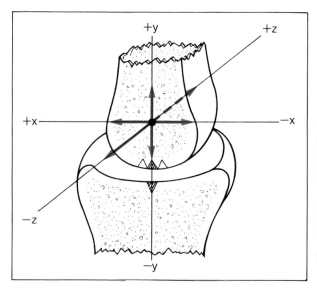

Figure **2** Translatory motion:
+y   traction      +x, −x  lateral gliding
−y   compression   +z, −z  anteroposterior gliding

- *Translatory Motion:* A joint or spinal segment can undergo to a small degree passive motion without an angular component being present.
  Separation of the joint surfaces is defined as traction, in contrast to movement of the joint surfaces against each other in a parallel plane, which is called gliding (Fig. **2**). Again translatory motion can also be defined as traction motion along three axes, i.e., x, y, z.
- *Joint Play:* The joint play is the sum of all passive angular and translatory motions (Fig. **3**). The endfeel associated with joint movement is of great diagnostic and therapeutic significance.
- *Physiologic Barrier:* Maximal active range of motion in a joint about one of the three major axes (three coordinate systems, x, y, z) (Fig. **4**).
- *Anatomic Motion Barrier:* Maximal passive range of motion in a joint about one of the three major axes, x, y, z (Fig. **4**). Movement beyond the anatomic barrier will always result in pathologic-structural changes.
- *Pathologic Motion Barrier:* Diminished active and passive motion secondary to pathologic processes. Segmental, peripheral-articular dysfunction (Fig. **5**) (Zurich Convention).
- *Hard Endfeel at the Barrier:* The motion is limited by articular-arthrotic changes. A hard endfeel may also be caused by sudden spasm such as may be encountered in a positive Lasègue test when examining for a ruptured lumbar disk (Fig. **6**).

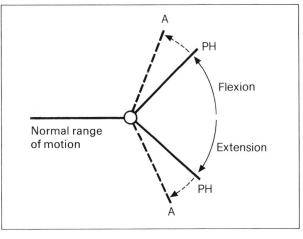

Figure **4**  Normal range of motion in a joint:
PH  physiologic barrier
A  anatomic motion barrier

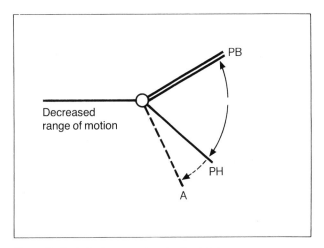

Figure **5**  Pathologic range of motion in a joint:
PB  pathologic motion barrier
A  anatomic motion barrier
PH  physiologic motion barrier

- *Soft Endfeel at the Barrier:* In this case motion is usually restricted by shortened tonic muscles, and occasionally by joint effusion (Fig. **7**).
- *Anatomic Position:* This is the position of the human body, standing erect with the palms of the hands turned forward and the arms at the side of the body, feet approximated and parallel. The patient looks straight ahead. Angle measurements are reported in reference to this anatomic position.
- *Present Neutral Position:* The present neutral position of a joint or spinal segment is that position in which joint play is greatest. Pathologic joint restriction and muscle imbalance result in changes of the present neutral position. Furthermore, the present neutral position is that position at which

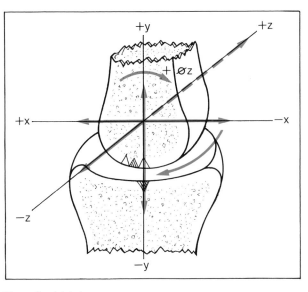

Figure **3**  Joint play:
+x, −x  laterale gliding
+z, −z  anteroposterior gliding
+y  traction
−y  compression
+Øz  rotation about the Z axis

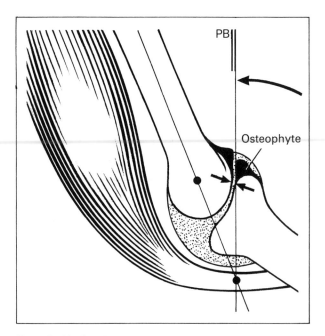

Figure **6**  Hard endfeel:
PB   pathologic motion barrier

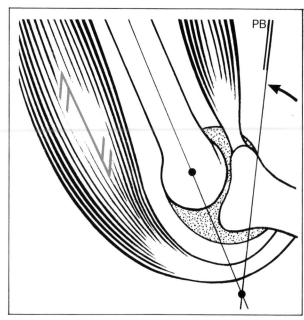

Figure **7**  Soft endfeel:
PB   pathologic motion barrier

the joint volume is greatest. Normally, pain intensity is smallest in the present neutral position.

– *Joint at the Barrier:* With the joint or spinal segment at the barrier, joint play is smallest. Joint stability is greatest in this position.

– *Treatment Plane of a Spinal Segment or Joint:* The treatment plane is perpendicular to the direction of traction. Gliding mobilization is effected in the treatment plane following the convex and concave rule.

– *Traction and Mobilization Levels* (Fig. **8**):
*Level I:* Minimal traction of magnitude sufficient to have zero pressure between the two joint surfaces.
*Level II:* Traction beyond level I without introducing stretch to the elastic structures, however.
*Level III:* The elastic structures are stretched to their respective physiologic barrier.
*Level IV:* Irreversible overstretch, rupture, or compression of ligaments, tendons, joint capsules, bones, or muscles, resulting in structural damage (distortions, luxations, fractures).

– *Convex Rule* (Fig. **9**): This rule applies to joints in which the distal joint partner has a convex joint surface. If angular movement is restricted due to changes in the joint itself, mobilization without impulse is utilized with the mobilization direction being opposite to that of the restricted mobility.

– *Concave Rule* (Fig. **10**): This refers to a joint in which the distal joint partner has a concave articu-

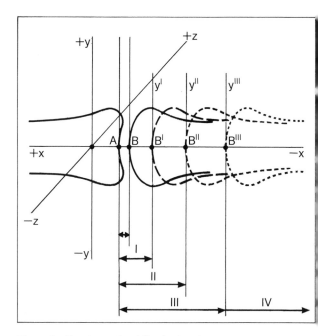

Figure **8**   Traction and mobilization levels:
AB    neutral position       AB‴  level III
AB′   level I                ABX  level IIII
AB″   level II

lar surface. If angular mobility is restricted due to canges in the joint itself, mobilization without impulse is used following the direction of joint restriction.

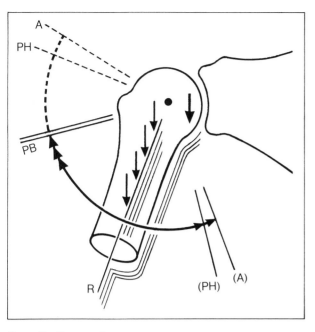

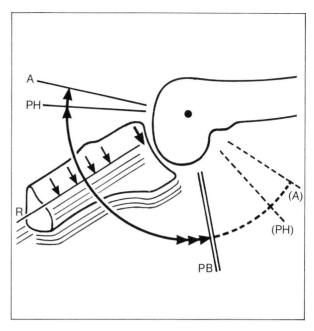

Figure **9**  Convex rule:
R    resting position (present neutral position)
PH   physiologic motion barrier
A    anatomic motion barrier
PB   pathologic motion barrier

Figure **10**  Concave rule:
R    resting position (present neutral position)
PH   physiologic motion barrier
A    anatomic motion barrier
PB   pathologic motion barrier

– Mobility Gain: This is defined as an increase in angular mobility secondary to stretching of the muscles. When a muscle spans two or more joints, it may be best to fix one joint while stretching the muscles over the other joint, which subsequently provides greater mobility to the stationary joint.
– *Provocative Testing* (Fig. **11**): Induced specific and well-localized mechanical stress to specific parts of the locomotor system may cause nociceptive reactions. These can both qualitatively and quantitatively change the patient's pain perception, change muscle tone or autonomic functions.

Some of the terms in manual medicine have taken on specific meanings, but differ as to the country in which they have been used. For instance, the terms "manipulation" and "mobilization," even though utilized in various countries, encompass different meaning in the individual country.

– *Manipulation:* In the United States, manipulation is a rather general term that refers to any therapeutic procedure in which the hands are used to treat the patient. In Europe, manipulation refers to what is described in the English language or according to American osteopathic terminology as "high velocity, low amplitude thrust."
– *Mobilization:* Mobilization is known in the United States as soft tissue and articulatory type of treat-

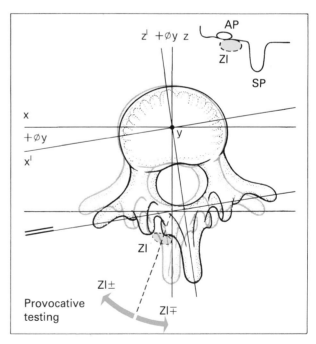

Figure **11**  Provocative tests: Quantitative changes at the zone of irritation:
ZI   zone of irritation
SP   spinus process
AP   articular pillar
PB   pathologic motion barrier
z–z' = $+\varnothing y$
x–x' = $+\varnothing y$

ment, including muscle energy techniques, whereas in Europe this term refers to the various types of articular mobilization without thrusting force.

- *Thrust or Impulse Techniques:* Both thrust and impulse describe the same entity, with thrust being preferred in the English language and impulse being more common in the European schools. In this text, the terms "mobilization with impulse" and "mobilization without impulse" were chosen, representing manipulative (thrust) and mobilizing procedures, respectively.

## 1.2 Treatment Techniques

- Mobilization without impulse
- Mobilization with impulse (the classic thrust techniques)
- Neuromuscular therapy (NMT)
  - NMT 1 (mobilization utilizing muscles directly)
  - NMT 2 (mobilization utilizing postisometric relaxation phase)
  - NMT 3 (mobilization utilizing reciprocal innervation)
- Home exercises
  - Muscle stretching
  - Autonomic mobilization
  - Isometric muscle strengthening exercises

### 1.2.1 Mobilization without Impulse

The following principles apply to mobilization techniques without impulse:

*Vertebral Column:*
- The spinal segments adjoining the restricted spinal segment are carried to their respective barriers (slack is taken up).
- The operator should make bony contact only with those structures that are located outside a zone of irritation.
- Mobilization is to be performed in the pain-free direction.
- The direction of mobilization is determined by the results obtained through provocative testing. Mobilization is in that direction in which the pain and nociceptive reactions are diminished.
- Duration of this mobilization technique ranges between 3 and 10 seconds.
- Traction may be used to improve pain (levels I–II), prior to applying the specific mobilization technique.
- To reduce pain, one may start with traction (mobilization level I–II).

- Mobilization of a peripheral joint should not lead to mobility beyond the anatomic barrier (mobilization level III).
- Mobilization should not mobilize a segment beyond its anatomic motion barrier (mobilization level III).

*Peripheral Joints:*
- The restricted joint is carried to its present neutral position.
- The hands are placed as close to the joint as possible, and in most instances the proximal joint partner is fixated, whereas the distal partner is mobilized.
- Mobilization direction is chosen according to the convex or concave rule leading to greater mobility in that particular joint.

The force-time diagram (Fig. **12**) demonstrates that minimal force is applied when positioning the patient. During the mobilization procedure, the force is increased gradually, and then it is gradually reduced (3–10 seconds).

As can be seen from the distance-time diagram (Fig. **13**) mobilization starts from the pathologic barrier, and the movement gained should not be beyond the anatomic motion barrier (Fig. **14**).

This procedure is repeated several times resulting in improved movement in the direction of the physiologic and anatomic motion barriers.

Mobilization procedures without impulse should be gentle and not painful to the patient.

### 1.2.2 Mobilization with Impulse (Manipulation, Classic Thrust Techniques)

The following considerations are important when applying the mobilization techniques with impulse:

*Vertebral Column:*
- Slack is taken up in the spinal segments adjoining the restricted joint (neighboring segments at their barriers).
- This procedure should not be painful to the patient.
- Manipulation (mobilization with impulse) is effected in the pain-free direction.
- The choice of direction for the mobilization with impulse is determined by the results from provocative testing. Mobilization is effected in that direction in which pain and nociceptive reactions are diminished (Fig. **11**).
- The impulse force should be of sufficient magnitude to introduce movement in the restricted joint, but not beyond the anatomic barrier (mobilization level III).

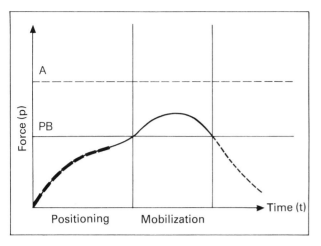

Figure **12** Force/time diagram for mobilization without impulse:
A    anatomic motion barrier    PB    pathologic motion barrier

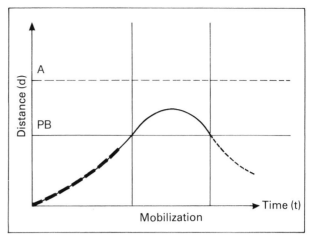

Figure **13** Distance/time diagram for mobilization without impulse:
A    anatomic motion barrier    PB    pathologic motion barrier

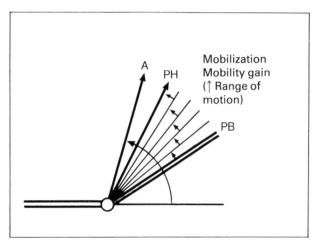

Figure **14** Mobilization without impulse/mobility gain:
A    anatomic motion barrier
PH    physiologic motion barrier
PB    pathologic motion barrier

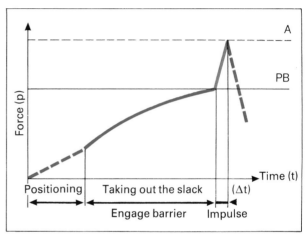

Figure **15** Force/time diagram for mobilization with impulse (thrust). Important is the short time Δt (high velocity):
A    anatomic motion barrier
PB    pathologic motion barrier

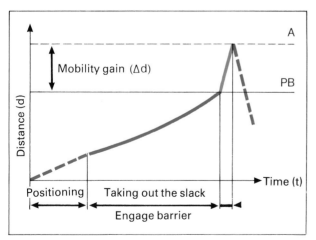

Figure **16** Distance/time diagram for mobilization with impulse (thrust). Important is the small amount of distance Δd (low amplitude):
A    anatomic motion barrier    PB    pathologic motion barrier

*Peripheral Joints:*
– The restricted joint is brought to its present neutral position.
– The operator places his hands close to the joint fixating the proximal joint partner. The impulse is normally perpendicular to the treatment plane.
– Manipulation treatment (mobilization with impulse) is from level II to mobilization level III.

The force/time diagram (Fig. **15**) demonstrates that minimal force only is applied during patient positioning. The distance/time diagram (Fig. **16**) shows that the force of impulse moves beyond the pathologic barrier but not beyond the anatomic barrier.

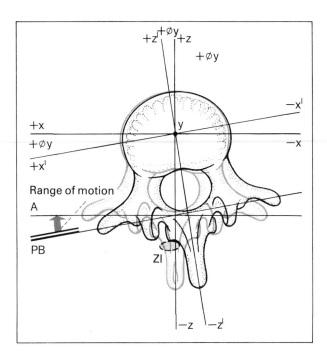

Figure **17**  Mobilization with impulse:
$z - z'$ = $+\emptyset y$
$x - x'$ = $+\emptyset y$
PB    pathologic motion barrier
A     anatomic motion barrier

The abdominal musculature introduces great flexion to the spinal column, which must be compensated for by the back extensor muscles. In regard to the neck muscles, one has to differentiate between postural and motion function. Strong muscles are necessary to stabilize the head in its position. Rotation of the head, to the left, for instance, is brought about by the action of the right transversospinal system, the sternocleidomastoid muscle, and the splenius capitis muscle on the left (again only the most important muscles are mentioned). Rotation restriction to the left can be caused by a shortened sternocleidomastoid on the left, or the rotator and multifidi muscles (Fig. **18**). It is thus important to examine each region of the spine with these concepts of functinal disturbance in mind, in order to be able to select the appropriate treatment procedure.

The impulse (manipulation, or thrust technique) is characterized by a high-velocity, low-amplitude force introduced beyond the pathologic barrier (Fig. **17**).

### 1.2.3  Neuromuscular Therapy

NMT includes treatment procedures that improve mobility and stretch muscles by utilizing direct muscle action as well as the associated neuromuscular reflex mechanisms (refer to Dvorak and Dvorak, Manual Medicine, Diagnostics).

A well-founded knowledge of the functional anatomy is indispensable for proper neuromuscular treatment. Concerning the spinal areas, it is important to know that rotation to one side is caused by the contralateral transversospinal system but may be limited by shortened ipsilateral transversospinal muscles, as well.

Trunk rotation is effected by muscles oblique or even perpendicular to the longitudinal axis of the vertebral column. This is primarily due to the action of the short and medium length transversospinal muscles, especially the rotator and multifidi muscles. Significant trunk rotation, however, requires the action of additional trunk muscles, such as those lateral abdominal muscles that connect the lateral aspect of the thorax with of pelvic crest on the opposite side.

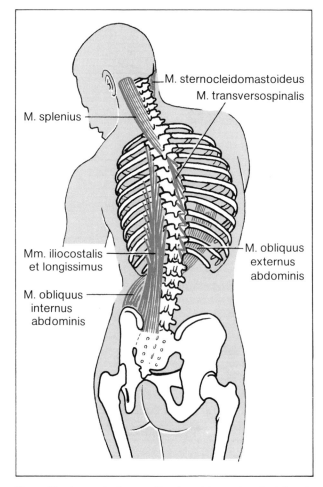

Figure **18**  Anatomic diagram: Rotation of the trunk to the left and the associated contracted muscles.

### 1.2.3.1 NMT 1: Mobilization utilizing Agonistic Muscles

Starting from the pathologic barrier, the patient effects mobilization by contracting the appropriate agonistic muscles which leads to movement beyond the pathologic barrier. The slack is taken up in the spinal segments next to the restricted joints. Since it is often difficult for the patient to learn these new movements, the operator can help both quantitatively and qualitatively by using palpatory assistance and verbal feedback to the patient.

NMT 1 teaches the patient those mobilization techniques that he often can perform on his own.

The following considerations are of significance when utilizing NMT 1:

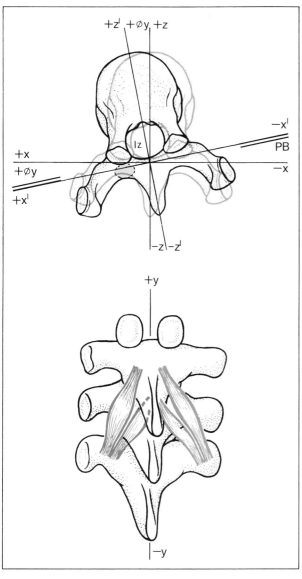
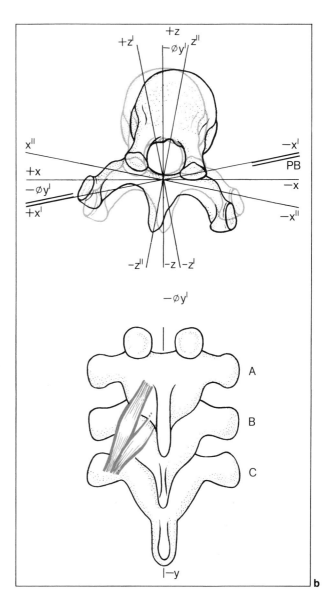

Figure **19**  NMT 1:
Red:  Agonistic muscles (rotater muscles), tonic muscles
Blue:  Antagonistic muscles (rotater muscles),
**a** conflict situation:
$$+z - (+z') = +\varnothing y$$
$$+x - (+x') = +\varnothing y$$
PB  pathologic motion barrier
ZI  zone of irritation

**b** mobilization step:
$$\left. \begin{array}{l} +x' - (+x'') = -\varnothing y' \\ +z' - (+z'') = -\varnothing y' \end{array} \right\} \text{ mobility gain}$$
A  mobilzed vertebra
B, C  fixed vertebrae
  Direction of mobilization

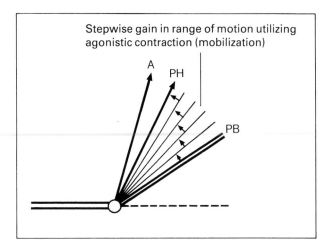

Figure **20**   NMT 1: Observe the stepwise mobility gain (increased range of motion) by repetitively contracting the agonistic muscles to the physiologic barrier:
A    anatomic motion barrier
PH   physiologic motion barrier
PB   pathological motion barrier

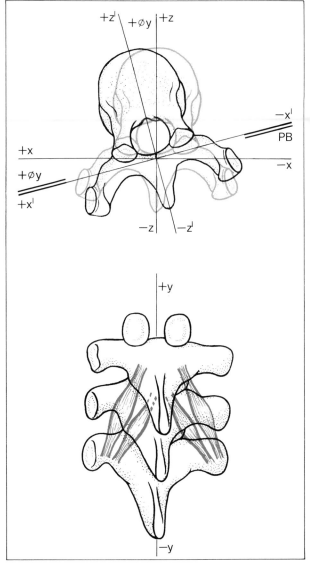

Figure **21a**

- The restricted joint must first be carried to its present pathologic barrier. The remainder of the spinal column: the segments distal to the restricted joints are fixated (slack is taken up) (Fig. **19a**).
- The patient introduces some movement beyond the pathologic motion barrier by contracting specific muscle groups (Fig. **19b**). Stepwise gain of movement (Fig. **20**).
- Duration of muscle contraction is between 2 and 5 seconds.
- Since this type of movement is often new to the patient and at times difficult to learn, it may be of benefit to use passive motion to guide the joint to the pathologic barrier.
- When teaching certain movements, it may be of benefit to stimulate by touch the cutaneous and muscular components in the area of those muscles that need to be contracted.
- This type of procedure is to be repeated several times in one session under supervision by the operator. The patient should also perform them several times on his own, on the same day.

### 1.2.3.2  NMT 2: Mobilization Utilizing Postisometric Relaxation of the Antagonists

If muscle testing reveals shortened tonic muscles, then there will always be diminished associated regional mobility, be it in the spinal areas or the peripheral joints (Fig. **21a**). Isometric contraction and subsequent stretching during the postisometric

relaxation phase may return the muscles often to their normal length. Muscle stretching mobilizes passively the corresponding joint or spinal segment. It can also be mobilized independently, however.

In many cases, however, there is weakening of the phasic muscles in addition to muscle shortening, and as a rule the muscles should be *stretched before strengthened*.

NMT 2 may be most beneficial in cases in which there is a soft endfeel with angular motion testing.

The following considerations are of significance when utilizing NMT 2:
- The incriminated muscle is stretched to near maximum and then optimal isometric contraction away

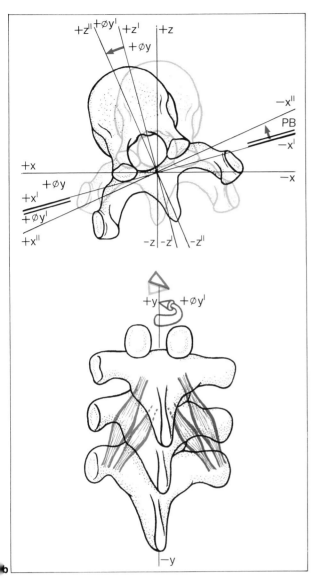

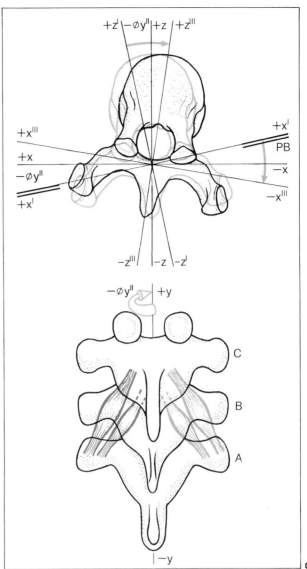

Figure **21** NMT 2 (i. e., rotation right $[-\varnothing y]$ is limited by shortening of the right transversospinal muscle system).

**a** conflict situation:

$+z - (+z') = +\varnothing y$
$+x - (+x') = +\varnothing y$

Red: Shortened rotation antagonistic muscles (rotator muscles)
Blue: Rotation agonistic muscles (rotator muscles)
PB  pathologic motion barrier

**b** Isometric contraction

$\left.\begin{array}{l} +z' - (+z'') = +\varnothing y' \\ +x' - (+x'') = +\varnothing y' \end{array}\right\}$ extent of isometric contraction

PB  pathologic motion barrier
    Resistance
    Direction of isometric contraction

**c** Mobilization step:

$\left.\begin{array}{l} +z' - (+z''') = -\varnothing y'' \\ +x' - (+x''') = -\varnothing y'' \end{array}\right\}$ gain in mobility

Blue: Rotation agonistic muscles (rotator muscles)
Yellow: Rotation agonistic muscles that provide stretch (rotator muscles)
A    fixed vertebra
B, C  mobilizing vertebra
PB   pathologic motion barrier

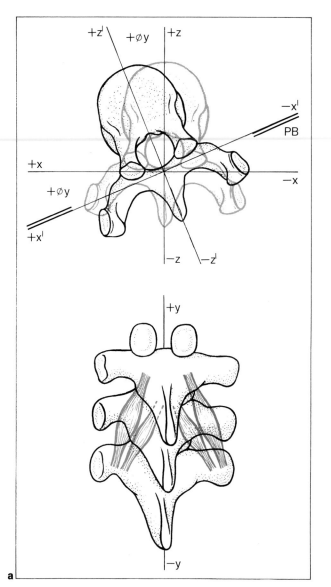 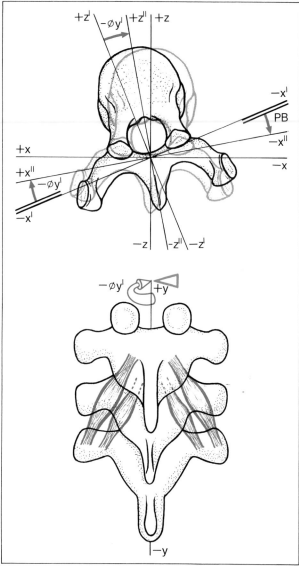

Figure **22**  NMT 3 (i. e., right axial rotation [$-\varnothing y$] is limited by shortening of the right transversospinal muscle system):

**a** Conflict situation:

$$\left.\begin{array}{l} +z - (+z') = +\varnothing y \\ +x - (+x') = +\varnothing y \end{array}\right\} \text{Motion restriction}$$

Red:   Shortened rotation antagonistic muscles (rotator muscles)
Blue:   Rotation agonistic muscles (rotator muscles)
PB      pathologic motion barrier

**b** Isometric Contraction:

$$\left.\begin{array}{l} +x' - (+x'') = -\varnothing y' \\ +z' - (+z'') = -\varnothing y' \end{array}\right\} \text{extent of isometric contraction}$$

Green:  Isometric contraction of the rotation agonistic muscles (rotator muscles)
             Direction of isometric contraction
             Resistance
PB       pathologic motion barrier

**c** Passive Mobilization:

$$\left.\begin{array}{l} +z'' - (+z''') = -\varnothing y'' \\ +x'' - (+x''') = -\varnothing y'' \end{array}\right\} \text{extent of passive mobilization}$$

             Mobilization direction beyond pathologic barrier
Yellow:  reciprocally inhibited rotation antagonistic muscles
Blue:    postisometrically relaxed rotation agonistic muscles

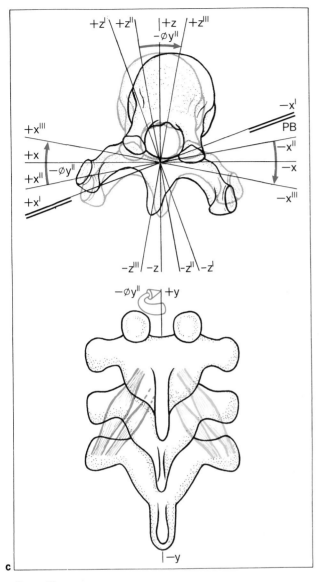

Figure **22 c**

### 1.2.3.3 NMT 3: Mobilization Utilizing Reciprocal Inhibition of the Antagonists

Isometric contraction is in the direction of motion restriction. The muscles antagonistic to those muscles that need to be relaxed are isometrically contracted, with the restricted joint being fixated. This is in contrast to NMT 1 in which the spinal segments adjoining the restricted joint are fixated. This technique is utilized when isometric contraction of the shortened tonic musculature is painful. This condition is often found with radicular syndromes.

The following considerations are of significance:
- The restricted spinal segment is carried to the pathologic barrier (Fig. **22a**).
- The restricted spinal segment or peripheral joint is fixated barring further movement.
- The first step of treatment includes pure isometric contraction in the direction of motion restriction (exact fixation/reciprocal inhibition). Duration of isometric contraction is between 5 and 10 seconds (Fig. **22b**).
- In the second step, careful passive mobilization is performed beyond the pathologic motion barrier (Figs. **22c, 23**). This mobilization requires significantly smaller forces than those applied with the stepwise stretching procedures during the postisometric relaxation phase of NMT 2.

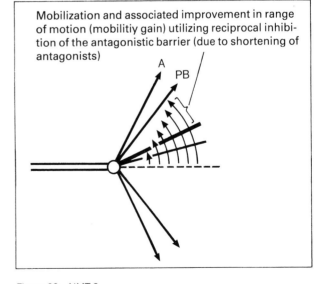

Figure **23**　NMT 3:
A　anatomic motion barrier
PB　physiologic motion barrier

from the pathologic barrier (Fig. **21b**) is introduced.
- The muscle is subsequently stretched for 3 to 10 seconds during the postisometric relaxation phase (Fig. **21c**).
- Stepwise stretching: starting from this new position, the muscle is again stretched maximally and isometrically.
- In most of the cases the patient needs to learn a stretching exercise program that he follows on a regular basis on his own at home (refer to "Home Exercise training").

# 2 Indications for Manual Therapy

Manual therapy concerns itself with the treatment of both functional disturbances in the spine or the extremity joints and abnormal muscle function, including the shortening, weakening, and imbalance of muscles.

With a good history and through a functional and palpatory examination of the locomotor system, one can utilize certain criteria that help one determine if and what manipulative treatment is indicated.

Criteria used for the indication of manual therapy include localized and referred pain, local soft tissue abnormalities, such as the zone of irritation, pathologic motion barrier (also referred to as motion restriction or hypomobility in the spinal segments, entire spinal regions, or the extremity joints), as well as muscular imbalance, be it regional (muscle shortening or weakening) or general (spondylogenic myotendinosis).

Optional criteria are muscular imbalance, both the regional type (muscle shortening and weakening) and the general type (spondylogenic myotendinosis), and a successful trial manual treatment attempt (Table 1).

The trial or provisional treatment attempt is of great importance, however. After the operator has eliminated possible contraindications, he will be able to make a provisional diagnosis and accordingly set up an appropriate treatment plan. With a trial manipulative treatment he can then evaluate whether or not the diagnosis and treatment procedure were correct. In cases in which there is neither subjective nor objective improvement seen with the provisional treatment procedure, and assuming that the chosen procedure had been executed correctly, a new diagnosis should be considered. Provisional or trial treatment is especially significant when dealing with muscular imbalance and mechanic joint disturbances. Using palpation as a diagnostic tool, a zone of irritation should improve with and during the trial treatment, both quantitatively and qualitatively. Tendinoses, in contrast, tend to improve only after a certain latent period, if at all.

The various criteria are further differentiated when choosing the individual treatment procedures or a combination thereof. Table 1 summarizes the criteria used and how they apply to the various treatment

Table 1   Indication for Manual Therapy

| | Treatment of | | | | |
| --- | --- | --- | --- | --- | --- |
| | Joints | | Muscles | | |
| | Mobilization with Impulse ("Thrust") | Mobilization without Impulse | Neuromuscular Therapy (NMT) | Stretching/ Strengthening | Home Exercise Training |
| Pain, acute | + + + | + | | | |
| Pain, chronic | + | + + | + + + | + + + | + + + |
| Pain, localized | + + + | + | | | |
| Pain, referred | + + | + + | + | + + + | + + |
| Segmental restriction with hard endfeel | + + + | + | | | |
| Segmental restriction with soft endfeel | | + + + | + + + | + + + | |
| Segmental restriction with pain | | + + + | + + + | + + + | |
| Segmental restriction without pain | + + + | + | + | + | |
| Segmental hypermobility | | | | + + + | + + + |
| Zone of irritation, prominent | + + + | + + | | | |
| Zone of irritation, discrete | | + | + + | | |
| Muscular imbalance, significant | | | + + + | + + + | + + + |
| Muscular imbalance, discrete | | | | | + + + |

modalities. This list, however, is not more than a mere guideline, because distinct borders are often absent. The more the operator is able to elicit a specific finding, the more he will be able to apply a specific and appropriate tratment procedure.

The choice of treatment procedure also depends on the onset and duration of the patient's pain, differentiating between an acute onset (0 to 14 days) and chronic pain (longer than 30 days). Again, there is no distinct border, but the time between days 14 and 30 can be described as a "subchronic" state. For simplicity reasons, the terms "acute" and "chronic" are used exclusively in this text. The patient can describe the pain as either localized or referred. The operator should pay particular attention to and differerentially analyze the patient's symptom complex, since there may be confounding spondylogenic of arthrogenic correlations coexisting. The typical pain along the course of a nerve root or that following a peripheral nerve root distribution should be viewed as the result of radicular compression.

Empirically, patients with acute and localized pain seem to respond better to mobilization with impulse (thrust) as long as the pathologic barrier had been engaged without difficulty during positioning. Patients with chronic or referred pain (as correlated with the spondylogenic reflex syndrome) should be treated by mobilization without impulse or neuromuscular therapy first.

The examination of joint mobility (large angular range of motion) and the evaluation of the joint play assess the three-dimensional range of motion and the extent of gliding movement in at least two directions. Furthermore, the evaluation of the endfeel is of equally great importance. A hard endfeel is associated with articular changes in the joint itself, whereas a soft endfeel is often due to shortened muscles, or, as in some instances, joint effusion. A reactive, sharp pain, as seen, for instance, with a positive Lasègue-test in the situation of a ruptured lumbar disk, or seen with cervical disk herniation, may also cause a hard endfeel.

The choice of treatment modality is dependent on the presence or absence of pain during the examination. Patients with pain-free segmental hypomobility and hard endfeel should be treated by mobilization with impulse (thrust). Patients with painful segmental hypomobility and soft endfeel should be treated by mobilization without impulse or neuromuscular therapy.

In the presence of hypermobility, both mobilization with and without impulse are contraindicated, whereas neuromuscular therapy may be partially applicable. Muscular imbalance in these patients must be improved. Stabilizing surgical procedures or orthotics may have to be considered, which requires careful evaluation.

Incidental findings such as quiescent, pain-free dysfunctions at the spine or the extremity joints should not be treated by mobilization. If there is also a muscular imbalance present, the patient should be encouraged to perform certain specific exercises at home, i.e., muscle stretching, self-mobilization, or isometric muscle strength training.

# 3    Patient Response to Manual Therapy

*The patient feels improvement after treatment:*
– Treatment is repeated until the patient is symptomfree or until the treatment goal has been attained.

*The patient's symptoms are exacerbated for hours subacutely after treatment but show improvement the day after treatment:*
– Continue treatment regimen.

*The patient's symptoms are exacerbated immediately after treatment:*
– The patient should be reassured.
– Soft traction of the treated spinal segments (along body axis), possibly soft massage of the paravertebral muscles.
– Local infiltration with local anesthetics.
– Reevaluation of the previous findings.
– Detailed documentation of the physical findings, including neurologic assessment and history.

*Progressively worsening symptoms (over days, weeks to months):*
– Manipulative treatment should be discontinued and medical treatment or local infiltration, etc., should be considered.
– Reevaluation of the previous diagnostic findings.
– Neurologic, rheumatologic, or orthopedic consultations may become necessary and should not be postponed.

*In case of neurologic complications:*
– Immediate hospitalization.
– Complete documentation of the incident and all findings (refer to "Complications").

*The patient's status remains unchanged, neither improvement nor worsening of the initial symptoms ("Sempre-lo-stesso-syndrome") after several treatment procedures (three to five treatments, maximum of eight treatments):*
– Discontinue treatment and reevaluate the patient's psychosocial situation.

# 4  Contraindications to Manual Therapy

- Acute inflammatory processes:
  - Absolute
  - Relative
- Destructive Processes, such as primary tumors or metastases
- Marked osteoporosis
- Significant degenerative changes
- Vertebral basilar insufficiency
- Radicular compression syndrome
- Deformities
- Whiplash injuries to the cervical spine
- Hypermobility
- Psychologic changes, such as neuroses, hysteria, depression

## Diagnosis: Acute Ruptured Lumbar Disk

| Mobilization with Impulse (Thrust) | Mobilization without Impulse | NMT Type 1 | NMT Type 2 | NMT Type 3 |
|---|---|---|---|---|
| Almost always, this technique is contra-indicated; if treatment is possibly attempted, the following criteria must be fulfilled: <br>- Relatively pain-free positioning is possible <br>- Prior trial treatment using mobilization without impulse was successful <br>- Other treatment modalities have been unsuccessful <br>- The patient is informed about the increased risk of this therapeutic procedure | Mobilization without impulse may be attempted when <br>- Relatively pain-free positioning is possible <br>- Mobilization does not exacerbate patient's symptoms | Nonadvisable in most of the cases because pain is exacerbated. Optimal isometric contraction beyond the pathologic barrier is often impossible secondary to excess pain | Stretching of the shortened tonic muscles is frequently beneficial. Muscle stretch should not lead to pull at the nerve root | This is often the only manipulative treatment possible in the acute state. Exact localization, and fixation become extremely important |

Rather than manipulative treatment, the major treatment modality of the acute or subacute ruptured lumbar disk, if not surgical, should be medical or supplemented by passive physical therapy. We refer to the standard texts regarding the indications for surgery or chemonucleolysis.

## Diagnosis: Acute Ruptured Cervical Disk

| Mobilization with Impulse (Thrust) | Mobilization without Impulse | NMT Type 1 | NMT Type 2 | NMT Type 3 |
| --- | --- | --- | --- | --- |
| Absolutely contraindicated in the cervical spine; there is great risk for spinal cord compression secondary to mass prolapse | Contraindicated in the cervical spine. In the chronic state treatment may be attempted if<br>– Patient positioning reduces the pain<br>– The mobilization technique does not exacerbate pain | Often nonbeneficial because optimum isometric contraction beyond the motion barrier is impossible due to significant pain | Stretching of the shortened muscles, in particular the suboccipital muscles, is often of benefit. Muscle stretching should not lead to tugging at the nerve roots | This may be the only manipulative treatment procedure applicable in the acute state. Exact fixation and localization and optimal isometric contractions are of paramount importance |

Treatment of the acute cervical ruptured cervical disk, if not surgical, should be primarily medical and supported by passive physical therapy much more so than manipulative therapy. As a rule, treatment should be initiated with NMT type 3. Mobilization without impulse should be applied extremely carefully, and the mobilizing forces should be applied appropriately carefully. Regarding indications for surgery, we refer to the standard texts.

## Diagnosis: Recent Soft Tissue Injury to the Cervical Spine
– No radiologic evidence of instability
– No neurologic deficits

| Mobilization with Impulse (Thrust) | Mobilization without Impulse | NMT Type 1 | NMT Type 2 | NMT Type 3 |
| --- | --- | --- | --- | --- |
| Mobilization procedures should not be applied in the first 4–6 weeks following an accident with major mechanical trauma | | After the acute phase (i.e., 4–6 weeks), the NMT type 1 technique may be well indicated for soft tissue treatment of the cervical spine if<br>– There is no segmental instability<br>– No relapses occur within hours of treatment | In the acute phase, NMT type 2 treatment is contraindicated unless, when applied, the technique would introduce maximal fixation to the affected area in the spine | NMT type 3 procedure can be utilized soon after the trauma as long as localization and fixation are specific |
| Mobilization with impulse may be applied if:<br>– Mobilization without impulse had been successful<br>– The operator is well experienced | If mobilization without impulse is to be used, the following points should be considered:<br>– NMT type 1 treatment was successful<br>– The mobilizing force is applied very carefully | | | |

In cases in which the cervical spine injuries were caused by major traumatic forces, rest, medical treatment and passive physical therapy are the more appropriate treatment modalities in the first 2–6 weeks.

When mobilization techniques bring about subjective or objective improvement of short duration only, one may be dealing with segmental instability in which case mobilization techniques would be contraindicated.

## Diagnosis: Chronic Phase of Soft Tissue Injury to the Cervical Spine

– No segmental instability
– No neurologic deficits

| Mobilization with Impulse (Thrust) | Mobilization without Impulse | NMT Type 1 | NMT Type 2 | NMT Type 3 |
|---|---|---|---|---|
| Mobilization techniques may prove to be beneficial, if:<br>– Prior trial treatment with NMT type 1 was successful<br>– Unequivocal segmental-regional findings(!)<br>– Patient positioning can be achieved without difficulty | Good for preparation to mobilization techniques with and without impulse as well as home training programs | The NMT type 2 procedure may assume great importance in cases of significant muscular imbalance | May be only necessary for acute exacerbations during the chronic phase |

Instability may be present if, soon after successful mobilization, relapses occurred. Functional radiographs may not be able to detect pathologic motion barriers because of muscle dysfunction and may be interpreted as normal thus preventing the diagnosis of instability.

Not rarely do signs and symptoms typical of soft tissue rheumatism develop when there has been soft tissue injury to the cervical spine ("fibrositis"). When this occurs, manipulative therapy should be chosen only with extreme caution because the patient may exaggerate psychologic disturbances (i.e., neurosis).

## Diagnosis: Cervical Vertigo (Including Cervical Migraine)

| Mobilization with Impulse (Thrust) | Mobilization without Impulse | NMT Type 1 | NMT Type 2 | NMT Type 3 |
|---|---|---|---|---|
| Mobilization procedures with and without impulse are indicated, if:<br>– The dysfunction is unequivocally segmental or regional<br>– Neurologic signs do not appear with provocative testing (positioning, palpatory pressure)<br>– Trial treatment using NMT type 1 is successful | A good technique for preliminary treatment and initiation of home exercise program | This may be an important technique especially in chronic situations in which there is pronounced muscle imbalance | This technique may be used in situations in which vertigo is exacerbated by different positioning. The reciprocal inhibition may be of benefit but exact localization and fixation are indispensable |

Evaluation of vertigo is often difficult. A specialist, who is familiar with functional disease of the cervical spine as well as neurologic and otologic disorders, will frequently have to be consulted.

Mobilization techniques and NMT type 1 techniques are absolutely contraindicated when the vertigo episodes are due to blood flow compromise in the vertebral basilar area.

## Diagnosis: Spondylolisthesis with Spondylolysis in the Lumbar Spine

| Mobilization with Impulse (Thrust) | Mobilization without Impulse | NMT Type 1 | NMT Type 2 | NMT Type 3 |
|---|---|---|---|---|
| Mobilization to the involved spinal segment is contraindicated. Neighboring segments and/or sacroiliac joints, however, should or must be treated by mobilization techniques | This is often of benefit for the neighboring spinal segments as well as the sacroiliac joint. Exact localization and fixation of the restricted joint are necessary | Muscle stretch techniques are frequently of great importance for spondylolisthesis treatment | This technique may be helpful in the acute phase so long as motion testing reveals a soft endfeel |

Manipulative therapy often concentrates on the segments neighboring those involved in the spondylolisthesis and rather supplements other treatment procedures, such as orthotics, stabilizing surgery. We refer to the standard texts of the orthopedic literature.

### Diagnosis: Bony Malformations in the Vertebral Column, Malformation of the Spinal Cord

| Mobilization with Impulse (Thrust) | Mobilization without Impulse | NMT Type 1 | NMT Type 2 | NMT Type 3 |
|---|---|---|---|---|
| | | | | |

Good orthopedic and neurologic knowledge is necessary to diagnose malformations in the spinal cord and the vertebral column. Together with functional pathologic findings, one is then able to determine if and which manipulative technique is indicated or contraindicated in the individual case.

### Diagnosis: Osteoporosis (with Pathologic Vertebral Fractures)

| Mobilization with Impulse (Thrust) | Mobilization without Impulse | NMT Type 1 | NMT Type 2 | NMT Type 3 |
|---|---|---|---|---|
| Both techniques are contraindicated as long as medical treatment has not brought about normalization of mineral content of the bones<br><br>Mobilization with impulse may be applicable, if:<br>– The mineral content of the bone is adequate<br>– Mobilization without impulse had been performed successfully<br>– Patient is informed in regard to the increased risk including that of possible rib or vertebral fractures | | This technique is contraindicated in the acute phase, whichever spinal area is affected. May be of benefit as trial treatment before mobilization without impulse | Stretching of the shortened tonic muscles is often necessary for postural physical therapy training or exercises to be successful | Often the only technique possible for acute fractures in the affected vertebral area |

Medical treatment is the major treatment modality in addition to passive physical therapy and orthotics at least in the acute fracture situation. In a chronic state manipulative therapy must be complemented by postural physical therapy training exercises. (For advanced osteoporosis without pathologic fractures, the same considerations apply.)

### Diagnosis: Ankylosing Spondylitis (Morbus Bechterew) – Acute Inflammatory State

| Mobilization with Impulse (Thrust) | Mobilization without Impulse | NMT Type 1 | NMT Type 2 | NMT Type 3 |
|---|---|---|---|---|
| This technique is absolutely contraindicated in the following regions:<br>– Sacroiliac joint<br>– Thorax regions, especially those that demonstrate acute exacerbation of inflammation | Mobilization without impulse and NMT type 1 procedures can be utilized to improve movement, but only if it is possible to guide the patient in a rather pain-free position and if mobilization does not lead to immediate or longer lasting exacerbation of the pain | | Muscular imbalance should be treated with NMT type 2 procedure even in the acute inflammatory state in order to prevent further deterioration of postural imbalance. The functional pathologic findings, however, must be unequivocal | This is a good technique to relax the patient, utilizing reciprocal inhibition |

Manipulative therapy should be applied very cautiously when dealing with inflammatory processes affecting the cervical spine. Segmental and regional instability in the atlanto-occipital joint must be excluded as well.

Analogous considerations apply for spondylopathy in association with psoriasis.

## Diagnosis: Ankylosing Spondylitis (Morbus Bechterew) without Clinical Signs of Acute Inflammation

| Mobilization with Impulse (Thrust) | Mobilization without Impulse | NMT Type 1 | NMT Type 2 | NMT Type 3 |
|---|---|---|---|---|
| Mobilization with impulse should only be applied if the trial treatment utilizing mobilization without impulse has proved successful | Successful trial treatment utilizing NMT type 1 is a good technique employed before mobilization without impulse is initiated | This technique is extremely effective and specific, especially when initiating the specific home exercise training | This technique is of great benefit when dealing with muscular imbalance of the tonic cervical spine muscles, muscles in the shoulder girdle, especially in cases in which there is progressive inflexibility of the thorax | Of insignificant importance only |

These techniques are absolutely contraindicated for spinal areas and the sacroiliac joint where bony growth has occurred. This is also true for hyperostotic spondylosis as well as spondylopathy in association with psoriasis.

## Diagnosis: Inflammation of the Vertebral Column in Association with Rheumatoid Arthritis

| Mobilization with Impulse (Thrust) | Mobilization without Impulse | NMT Type 1 | NMT Type 2 | NMT Type 3 |
|---|---|---|---|---|
|  |  |  |  |  |

If the cervical spine is affected, mobilizing techniques should be applied only in very rare instances and then with great caution. If there is atlantoaxial instability suspected or proved either clinically or radiologically, manipulative treatment to this region is absolutely contraindicated.

## Diagnosis: Abnormal Segmental or Regional Spinal Hypermobility (Congenital or Acquired)

| Mobilization with Impulse (Thrust) | Mobilization without Impulse | NMT Type 1 | NMT Type 2 | NMT Type 3 |
|---|---|---|---|---|
| Mobilization techniques and NMT type 1 techniques are contraindicated. Occasionally, mobilization techniques may be of benefit in the acute segmental or regional motion restriction state (with soft endfeel). In these situations, however, mobilizing force, as well as total number of treatments, should be minimal | | | NMT type 2 techniques are often indispensable for treatment of muscular imbalance or before stabilizing exercise training programs can be started | NMT type 3 utilizing reciprocal inhibition is well suited for regional relaxation therapy. These techniques should be supplemented by stabilizing exercise training therapy |

# 5    Manual Therapy

## Documentation of Examination Results

The following is a scheme for documenting pathological findings, including:
– direction of motion
– restriction of motion
– muscle shortening
– muscle weakening
– pain

| | | | |
|---|---|---|---|
| In | Inclination | El | Elevation |
| Rc | Reclination | IR | Internal Rotation |
| F | Flexion | ER | External Rotation |
| E | Extension | Ab | Abduction |
| SB | Side-bending | Ad | Adduction |
| R | Rotation | | |
| r | to the right | UD | Ulnar Abduction |
| l | to the left | RD | Radius Abduction |
| | | S | Supination |
| N | Nutation | P | Pronation |
| f | in flexing direction | | |
| e | in extending direction | | |

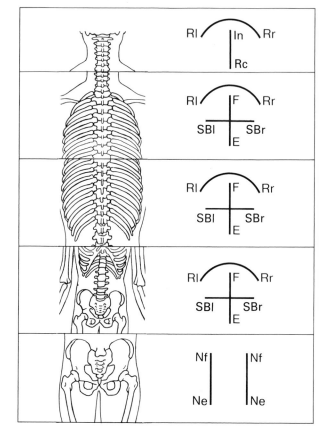

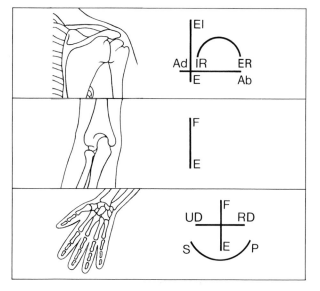

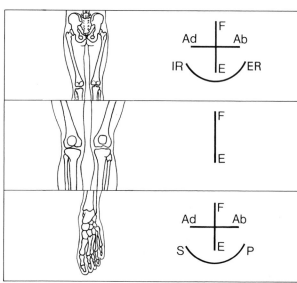

| Signs for Restriction of Motion: | |
|---|---|
| Normal range of motion | |
| Slightly restricted | |
| Very restricted | |
| Almost completely restricted (and akylosis) | |
| Pain at end of motion | |
| **Signs for Shortened Muscles:** (from origin to insertion) | |
| Slight shortening | |
| Marked shortening | |
| Extreme shortening | |
| **Signs for Weakened Muscles:** (origin to insertion) | |
| Slightly weak | |
| Very weak | |
| Extremely weak | |
| **Signs for Pain:** | |
| Localized or diffused pain | |
| Radiating pain | |
| Zone of irriation | |

| | | |
|---|---|---|
| NMT 1 | – Isometric Contraction<br>– Mobilization Direction | |
| NMT 2 | – Isometric Contraction | |
| | – Direction of Stretching | |
| NMT 3 | – Isometric Contraction | |
| | – Mobilization Direction | |
| Mobilisation without Impulse | – Mobilization Direction | |
| Mobilization with Impulse | – Mobilization Direction | |
| Point of Fixation | – Operator | |
| Point of Fixation | – Patient | |
| Resistance | – against isometric Barrier | |

23

# C0 to C1

## Mobilization without Impulse: Inclination-Reclination Restriction

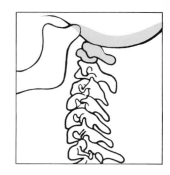

### Indication (Fig. a)

*Zone of irritation:* C0–C1.

*Motion testing:* Inclination-reclination restriction with hard endfeel.

*Pain:* Acute or chronic; suboccipital; pain may radiate toward the occiput and the region between the scapulae.

*Muscle testing:* Shortened suboccipital muscles.

*Autonomic symptoms:* Nonsystematic vertigo, exacerbated by palpatory pressure.

### Positioning

- Patient is sitting.
- The cervical spine is carried to its anatomic neutral or present neutral position.
- The restricted spinal segment is brought to the pathologic barrier.
- C2 is fixated at the articular pillars by the operator's thumb and index finger.
- The patient's head is fixated at the temporal regions (Fig. **b**).

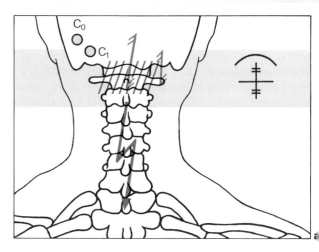

### Treatment Procedure

- Passive mobilization to improve inclination-reclination movement (Fig. **b**).

*Note:* During reclination, there is a gliding motion in an interior direction, whereas during inclination the gliding motion is in the posterior direction.

### Remarks

This mobilization technique is well suited to prepare the patient for inclination-reclination movement introduced with appropriate NMT procedures as well as self-mobilization techniques. If during or after the mobilization procedure vertigo appears, it may be due to one or a combination of the following:
- Mobilization was too forceful,
- Palpatory pressure was too hard over the zone of irritation,
- Atlantoaxial instability (primary chronic polyarthritis, post-traumatic)

If it is difficult to use this technique, one should first resort to NMT 2 or mobilization with impulse techniques.

Naturally, it is important to know what the contraindications are when using the impulse technique.

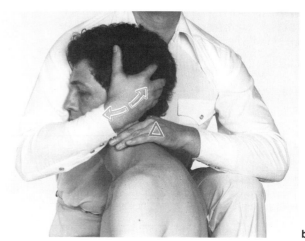

# C0 to C3

## Mobilization without Impulse: Axial Tractions

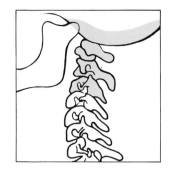

### Indication (Fig. a)

*Zone of irritation:* C0, C1, C2, C3, exacerbated by palpatory pressure.

*Motion testing:* Painful, restricted motion with segmental hypomobility and hard reflexogenic end-feel.

*Pain:* Acute in the neck region; worse with movement.

### Positioning

- Patient is sitting.
- The spinal segments C0 to C3 are brought to their present neutral position.
- C3 to T3 are flexed and "locked" in that position.
- With elbows resting on the patient's shoulders, the operator places both hands flat over the side of the patient's head.

*Note:* It is important that the present neutral position of the upper cervical spine is found first.

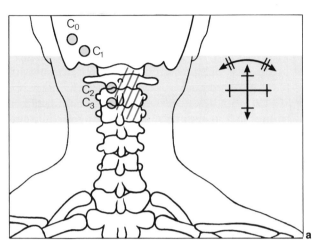

### Treatment Procedure

- Passive traction is introduced.
- Traction is started synchronously with the beginning of deep exhalation.
- The tractional force is slowly increased as the patient continues to breathe regularly and deeply.
- The tractional force is then slowly and carefully diminished (Fig. **b**).

*Note:* Forced respiration is to be avoided.

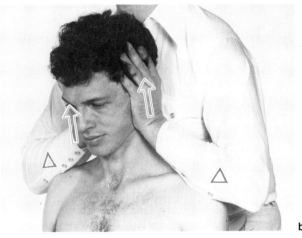

### Remarks

With the proper diagnosis and correct treatment procedure, the patient's pain should diminish both during and after the treatment. This traction procedure involves minimal risk to the patient.

# C1 to C2

## Mobilization without Impulse: Rotation Restriction

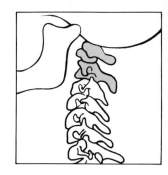

### Indication (Fig. a)

*Zone of irritation:* C1–C2

*Motion testing:* C1–C2 segmental rotation restriction, occasional inclination-reclination restriction with hard or soft endfeel.

*Pain:* Pain can be either acute or chronic. Localized to the neck region, may be radiating to the temporal area as well as the region between the scapulae.

*Muscle testing:* The levator scapulae or the descending portion of the trapezius muscle, or both, may be shortened.

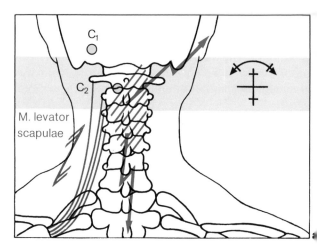

### Positioning

- Patient is sitting.
- The operator places his thumb and index finger over the articular processes of C2, thereby fixating the vertebra (Fig. **b**).
- The operator embraces the patient's head with his arm, so that he can place his small finger and the metacarpal bone of the small finger over the occiput and C1.
- The cervical spine is carried to its present neutral position.
- The incriminated segment is guided to its pathologic barrier.

### Treatment Procedure

- Passive mobilization to improve rotation is introduced, while the patient is asked to simultaneously direct his gaze in the direction of rotation movement (Fig. **c**).

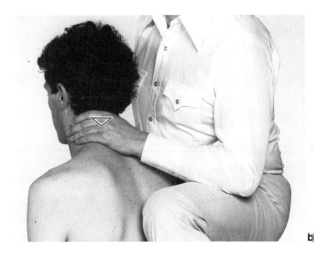

### Remarks

The individual mobilization step is rather small. Some traction should be applied to the cervical spine along with this mobilization technique.

Excessive force must be avoided because it could cause compression of the vertebral artery. If vertigo appears, the treatment must be terminated immediately.

If vertigo becomes apparent during the patient positioning phase, NMT-2 for the levator scapulae muscle or descending portion of the trapezius muscle should be employed instead.

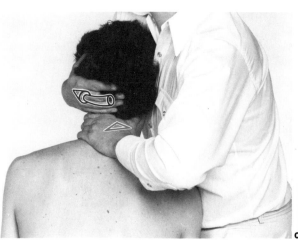

## Mobilization with Impulse (Thrust): Reclination Restriction

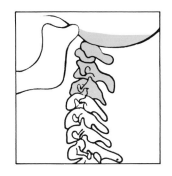

### Indication (Fig. a)

*Zone of irritation:* C0, C1, C2, C3.
*Motion testing:* Segmental reclination restriction with
hard endfeel.
*Pain:* Suboccipital area.

### Positioning

– Patient is supine. The operator places the proximal
phalanx of his index finger over the mastoid on the
restricted side.
– The other hand cradles the patient's chin, with the
forearm supporting the patient's temporal region
(Fig. **b**).
– The cervical spine is somewhat reclined/-extended
and side bent, which is coupled to a rotation
movement in this segment (forced rotation of the
axis, coupling motions in the cervical spine, please
refer to *Manual Medicine – Diagnostics*, p. 8).

### Treatment Procedure

This passive mobilization procedure utilizes a
superiorly directed impulse along the sagittal angle of
the joint inclinations. The force of impulse is directed
toward the patient's mastoid process (Fig. **b**).

### Remarks:

One should avoid greater than normal axis rotation because the
vertebral artery may otherwise be compromised in the craniocervical junction.

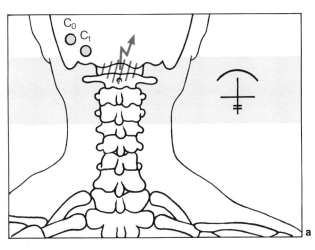

a

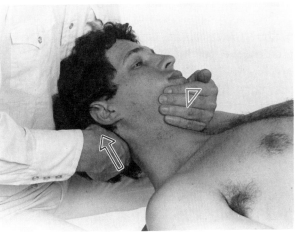

b

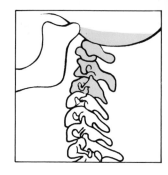

## Mobilization with Impulse (Thrust): Traction

### Indication (Fig. a)

*Zone of irritation:* C0, C1, C2, C3.
*Motion testing:* Segmental motion restriction with hard or soft endfeel.
*Pain:* Localized; radiating toward the occiput and to the region between the scapulae.

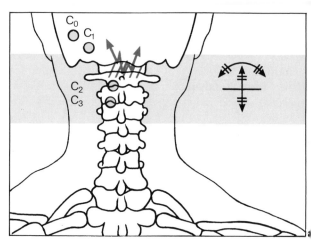

### Positioning

- The operator stands behind the seated patient, placing his thumb over the arch of the atlas, thereby creating a fulcrum (Fig. **b**).
- The operator then reaches around the patient's chin and head, aligning the patient's nose, chin, and elbow all in one plane (Fig. **c**).
- By rotating his trunk, the operator carries the patient's cervical spine to the pathologic barrier. Passive rotation as well as axial traction are introduced.

### Treatment Procedure

A superiorly directed impulse is effected through the operator's arm that cradles the patient's chin and head. There should be no extension introduced to the cervical spine, however (Fig. **d**).

### Remarks

Passive maximal rotation in the craniocervical junction may adversely affect the vertebral artery, and one must pay attention to the following two points:
- The patient should be totally relaxed
- The operator must be experienced in this technique (please refer to complications of manipulative therapy).

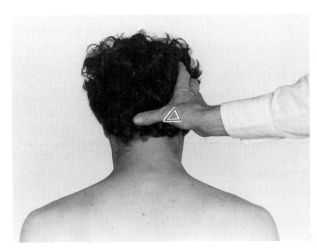

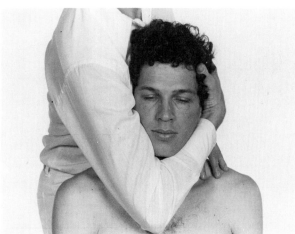

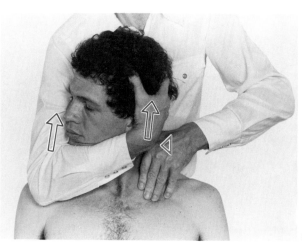

d

## Mobilization with Impulse (Thrust): Traction

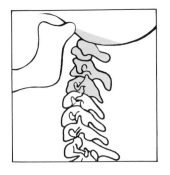

### Indication (Fig. a)

*Zone of irritation:* C0, C1, C2, C3.

*Motion testing:* Regional motion restriction with hard endfeel.

*Pain:* Acute; localized or radiating to the occiput area.

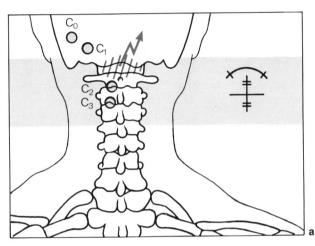

### Positioning

- The operator, standing behind the patient, places his hands flat over the patient's head in the parietal regions.
- He carefully rests his forearms on the patient's shoulders (Fig. **b**).
- Passive inclination is introduced to C0–C2.

### Treatment Procedure

- Traction along the body's axis is performed.
- When the patient is relaxed, one may introduce a superiorly directed impulse (thrust).

### Remarks

Please see also mobilization with impulse: Traction; patient supine (p. 27).

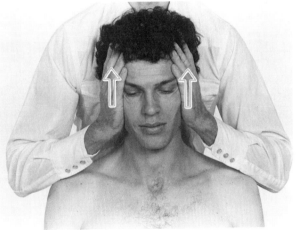

## Mobilization with Impulse (Thrust): Traction

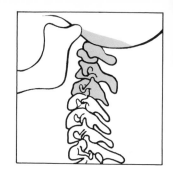

### Indication (Fig. a)

*Zone of irritation:* C0, C1, C2, C3.
*Motion testing:* Regional motion restriction with hard endfeel.
*Pain:* Acute; localized or radiating toward the occiput.

### Positioning

– Patient is supine.
– The patient's head is beyond the examination table resting in its normal anatomic or present neutral position on the thigh of the operator, who is seated behind the patient.
– The thumb and index finger of one hand are placed around the occiput, while the opposite hand cradles the patient's chin.
– Passive inclination of C0 to C2 is introduced (Fig. **b**).

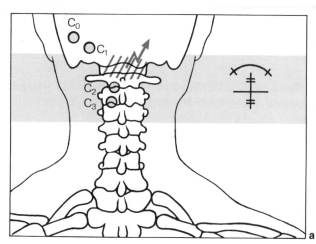

### Treatment Procedure

Traction in a superior direction along the body's axis. When the patient is relaxed, a superiorly directed impulse may be applied (Fig. **b**).

### Remarks

Traction is primarily directed toward the segments between C0 and C3 but can also be applied to spinal segments of the lower cervical spine.
This is a valuable technique for the rather anxious patient with acute neck pain.
In the patient with torticollis it is important that the present neutral position of the head be determined.

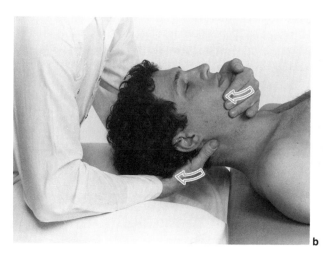

## Mobilization with Impulse (Thrust): Rotation Restriction

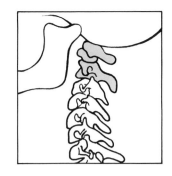

### Indication (Fig. a)

*Zone of irritation:* C1–C2.
*Motion testing:* Rotation restriction with hard end-feel.
*Pain:* Suboccipital area; occasionally radiating to the region between the scapulae.

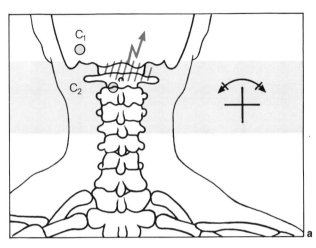

### Positioning

– Patient is supine, with his head resting on the thigh of the operator, who is seated behind the patient.
– The operator places the proximal phalanx of the index finger of the mobilizing hand over the transverse process of the atlas on the restricted side. His other hand fixates the patient's chin (Fig. **b**).
– The C1–C2 segment is brought to the pathologic motion barrier by introducing passive rotation, side-bending, and inclination.

### Treatment Procedure

A rotatory impulse force is directed toward the transverse process of the atlas (Fig. **b**).

### Remarks

The impulse should not contain a reclination component because the vertebral artery may otherwise be adversely affected.

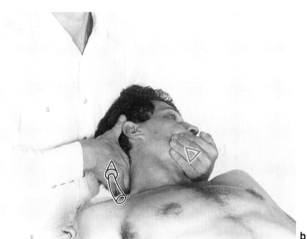

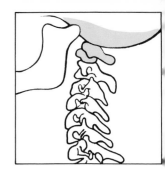

## NMT 1 and Self-Mobilization: Inclination-Reclination Restriction

### Indication (Fig. a)

*Zone of irritation:* C0–C1.

*Motion testing:* Segmental inclination-reclination restriction with hard or soft endfeel.

*Pain:* Chronic; occasionally radiating to the occiput and between the shoulder blades.

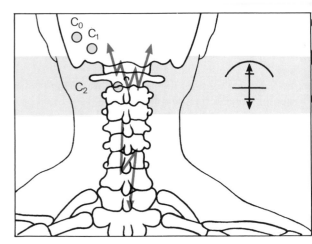

### Positioning

- Patient is seated.
- The cervical spine is in the present neutral position.
- NMT 1: the spinal segment is softly fixated at the articular pillars of C1 by the operator's fingers (Fig. **b**).

Self-mobilization: C1 is fixated with the small fingers. The remaining fingers and the thumb are placed flat over the remaining cervical spinal segments. The fingers are *not* bent behind the neck but rather placed flat on top of each other in order to avoid undue anterior traction (Fig. **c**).

- The spinal segment is carried to its pathologic barrier.

*Note:* Fixation must under all circumstances be soft. In the case of self-stabilization, one should apply only minimal anterior traction.

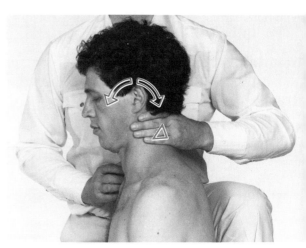

### Treatment Procedure

Active mobilization is applied to improve the inclination-reclination movement.

The inclination movement is performed during exhalation and with the patient looking toward the floor, whereas the reclination movement is executed during inhalation with the patient looking toward the ceiling (Fig. **b**).

### Remarks:

If vertigo appears during or after mobilization, the following causes may be incriminated:
- Too forceful a palpation at the zone of irritation.
- Excessive anterior traction during fixation.
- The procedure is done too quickly (hyperventilation?)
- Atlantoaxial instability (primary chronic polyarthritis or post-traumatic state).

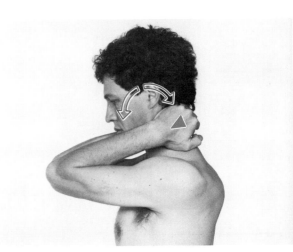

## NMT 1 and Self-Mobilization: Rotation Restriction

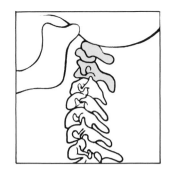

### Indication (Fig. a)

*Zone of irritation:* C1–C2.

*Motion testing:* Segmental rotation restriction with hard or soft endfeel.

*Pain:* Either acute or chronic; radiating to the occiput, temporal regions, or between the shoulder blades.

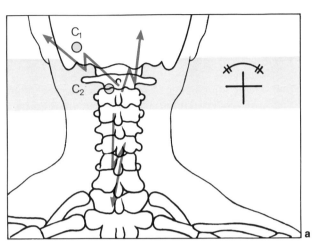

### Positioning

- The patient is seated.
- The cervical spine is carried to its anatomic position or present neutral position.
- NMT 1: The articular pillars of C2 are fixated with two fingers (Fig. **b**).

Self-mobilization: The operator's hypothenar eminence fixates the C2 articular pillar on the involved side (Fig. **c**).

- The spinal segment is carried to its pathologic barrier.

*Note:* The fingers should be placed gently over the articular pillars in order to diminish the chance of vertigo or pain.

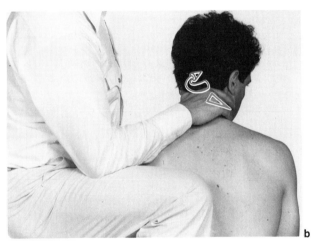

### Treatment Procedure

- Active mobilization is utilized in order to improve rotation.
- Step-by-step, the patient moves beyond the pathologic barrier whereby his gaze is directed toward the side of rotation (Fig.**5**).

*Note:* Jerky, abrupt to and fro movements should be avoided.

### Remarks

The path gained with each individual mobilization step is rather small.

If vertigo appears during mobilization, NMT 3 should be used, or in place of self-mobilization one should resort to NMT 2 for the descending portion of the trapezius muscle.

Possible causes of vertigo that must be exluded before one can proceed to an alternative treatment include:

- Too forceful a mobilization
- Instability
- Too great a pressure in the zone of irritation

If this technique causes other problems, mobilization with impulse techniques may be utilized. One should, however, be aware of the indications and contraindicatious for the specific treatment.

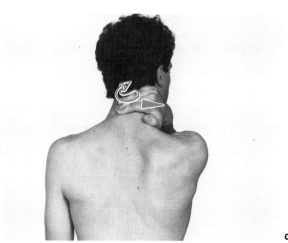

## NMT 2: Rotation Restriction

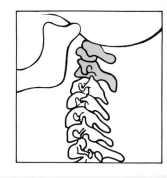

### Indication (Fig. a)

*Zone of irritation:* C1–C2.

*Motion testing:* Segmental rotation restriction with soft endfeel.

*Pain:* Acute or chronic. Localized to neck region, occasionally radiating to the occiput, temporal region, or between the shoulder blades.

*Muscle testing:* The suboccipital muscles are shortened.

*Autonomic symptoms:* Nonsystematic vertigo, exacerbated when pressure is applied.

### Positioning

- The patient is seated. The cervical spine is brought to its anatomic position or to present neutral position.
- The articular pillars of C2 are fixated by two fingers in a vise like manner.
- The operator, standing on the side to which the segment is to be mobilized, braces the patient's head (Fig. **b**).
- The cervical spine should neither be compressed nor side-bent.
- The spinal segment is brought to its pathologic barrier (Fig. **c**).

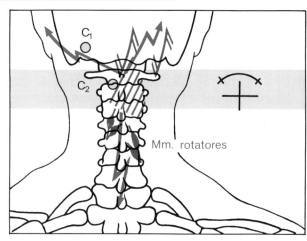

Mm. rotatores

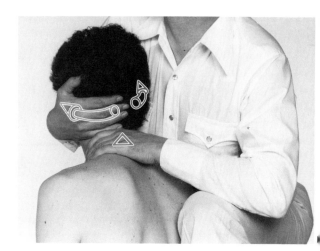

## NMT 2: Rotation Restriction (cont'd.)

### Treatment Procedure

– Maximal isometric contraction away from the pathologic barrier (Fig. **b, d**).
– During the postisometric relaxation phase and without releasing the fixating force, the head and neck are passively rotated beyond the pathologic barrier (Fig. **b, e**).

### Remarks

The path gained with each individual mobilization step is rather small. This technique is particularly well suited when there is motion restriction with soft endfeel.

If vertigo appears during or after treatment, one should consider the following possible causes:
– Undue pressure over the zone of irritation
– Forceful mobilization during the postisometric relaxation phase.

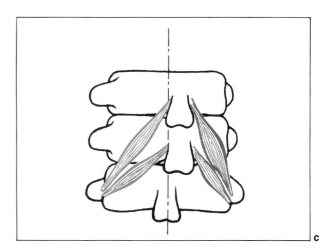

c

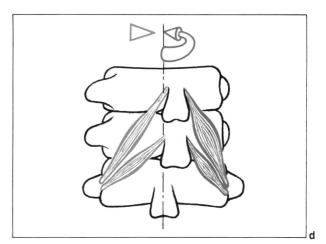

d

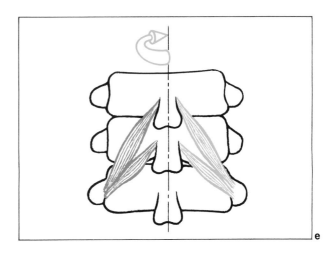

e

# C0 to C3

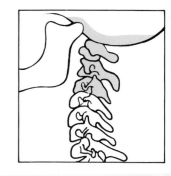

## NMT 2: Inclination Restriction

### Indication (Fig. a)

*Zone of irritation:* C0, C1, C2, C3.

*Motion testing:* Inclination restriction with soft end-feel.

*Pain:* Chronic; radiating toward the occiput and between the shoulder blades.

*Muscle testing:* Shortening of the rectus capitis, obliquus capitis, and the semispinalis capitis muscles. Often there is concurrent shortening in the descending portion of the trapezius and levator scapulae muscles and weakening of the muscles holding the shoulder blade to the thorax.

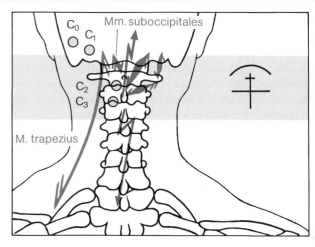

### Positioning

- The patient is supine
- The patient's shoulders rest on the examination table.
- The operator carefully fixates with two fingers the articular pillar and spinous process of C3.
- The head is embraced in such a manner that the patient's forehead rests against the operator's pectoral region.
- The hand is placed broadly over the occiput (Fig. **b**).
- The spinal segments C0 to C3 are brought to their respective pathologic barriers.

### Treatment Procedure

- The spine is isometrically extended during inhalation and the patient is asked to turn his eyes upward simultaneously.
- During exhalation, the spine is passively flexed and the patient is asked to look downward. The operator carefully follows the flexion movement with his hand and shoulder (Fig. **b**).

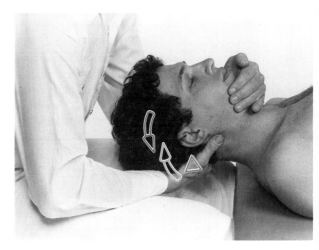

### Remarks

The patient should breath properly.
This technique cannot be used when there is hard endfeel with inclination (flexion) restriction.

## Mobilization without Impulse: Rotation Restriction

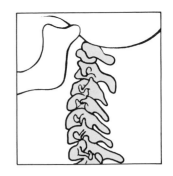

### Indication (Fig. a)

*Zone of irritation:* C2, C3, C4, C5, C6, C7, T1, T2, T3.

*Motion testing:* Segmental or regional rotation and/or side-bending restriction; hard endfeel.

*Pain:* Chronic; the neck region. Occasionally radiating to the shoulders, arms, occiput, and between the shoulder blades.

*Muscle testing:* Shortening of the descending portion of the trapezius and levator scapulae muscles, and weakening of the muscles that hold the shoulder blade in place.

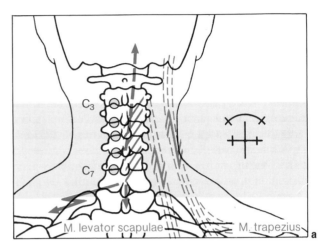

M. levator scapulae     M. trapezius     a

### Positioning

- The patient is seated.
- The cervical spine is brought to its anatomic position or the present neutral position.
- The vertebra below the involved spinal segment is fixated by the operator placing two fingers over the articular pillars (Fig.**b**).
- The involved spinal segment is carried to its pathologic barrier.

### Treatment Procedure

- Passive mobilization is effected by the small finger pulling in a rotational manner at the articular pillar of the superior vertebra of that segment. This rotation then is transmitted to the cervical spine above the involved spinal segment.
- The other hand, the mobilizing hand, introduces slight traction (Fig. **b**).

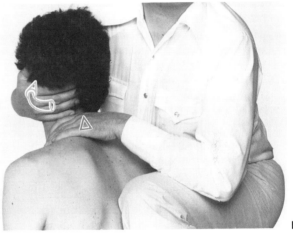

b

*Note:* The path gained with each mobilization is rather small.

### Remarks

In cases of radicular cervical syndromes, this technique may be utilized when superior traction is also introduced simultaneously. Radicular pain, however, must not worsen with this mobilization procedure.

If localized pain becomes apparent during the treatment, one should exclude the following possible causes.

- Too forceful a mobilization
- Excessive pressure over the zone of irritation

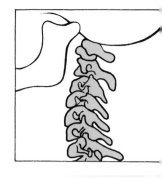

## Mobilization with Impulse (Thrust): Rotation Restriction

### Indication (Fig. a)

*Zone of irritation:* C2, C3, C4, C5, C6, C7, T1, T2, T3.

*Motion testing:* Segmental or regional rotation restriction with hard endfeel.

*Pain:* Diffuse distribution in the neck region; occasionally pain radiates in a pseudoradicular fashion to the arms and the region between the scapulae.

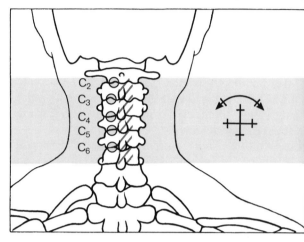

### Positioning

– Patient is supine. The operator places the proximal phalanx of his index finger over the transverse process of the vertebra above the segment that is to be mobilized.
– With his other hand, he cradles the patient's chin, while the head comes to rest on his forearm (Fig. **b**).
– The affected spinal segment is passively rotated and brought to its pathologic barrier.

### Treatment Procedure

– Slight traction is introduced to the entire cervical spine.
– The direction of the impulse is along the path of rotation and side-bending, which are the physiologic motion components in that segment (Fig. **b**).

### Remarks

The mobilizing force is also transmitted to the more inferior cervical spinal segments, with the intensity diminishing from superior to inferior.

This technique may compromise the vertebral artery, and thus careful and exact treatment execution is necessary.

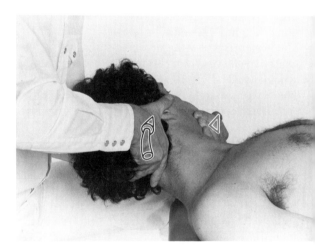

# C2 to T3

## Mobilization with Impulse (Thrust): Rotation Restriction

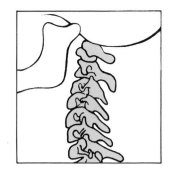

### Indication (Fig. a)

*Zone of irritation:* C2, C3, C4, C5, C6, T1, T2, T3.
*Motion testing:* Segmental rotation restriction with hard endfeel.
*Pain:* Localized; occasional pseudoradicular radiation to the arms or the region between the scapulae.

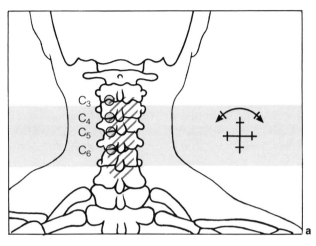

a

### Positioning

– Patient is sitting.
– The operator places his second metacarpal bone over the articular pillar of the vertebra below the spinal segment that is to be mobilized.
– With his other arm, he embraces the head in the tempero-occipital region and places the hypothenar and small finger over the vertebra above the spinal segment that is to be mobilized.
– Passive rotation is introduced from superior, bringing the incriminated spinal segment to the pathologic barrier.

### Treatment Procedure

– A rotatory impulse force is directed toward the vertebra below the restricted spinal segment in a superior direction at an angle of 15°.
– The impulse is introduced during exhalation (Fig. **b**).

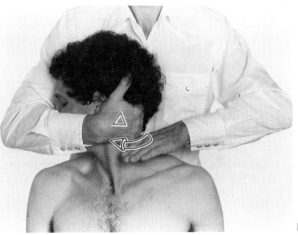

b

### Remarks

This is the technique of choice for problems in the midcervical spine.
One should note:
– The patient should be totally relaxed,
– The operator should be very familiar with this technique

# C2 to T3

## Mobilization with Impulse (Thrust): Rotation Restriction

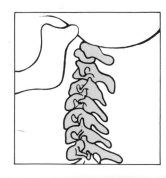

### Indication (Fig. a)

*Zone of irritation:* C2, C3, C4, C5, C6, C7, T1, T2, T3.

*Motion testing:* Segmental rotation restriction with hard endfeel.

*Pain:* Localized; occasionally radiating into the arms or the region between the shoulder blades.

### Positioning:

- Patient is sitting.
- The operator cradles the patient's head with his hand and forearm. The hypothenar and the small finger are placed over the articular pillar of the vertebra that lies above the involved spinal segment.
- The second metacarpal bone and the thumb of the other hand are placed over the articular pillar of the vertebra that lies below the involved spinal segment.
- Passive rotation of the head is introduced until the pathologic barrier of the restricted spinal segment is engaged (Fig. **b**).

### Treatment Procedure

- The rotatory impulse is directed toward the vertebra that adjoins superiorly the restricted spinal segment and is introduced while the patient exhales (Fig. **b**).

### Remarks

This is quite an effective technique, especially for the midthoracic spine. However, it should only be performed by persons who have great experience with this technique.

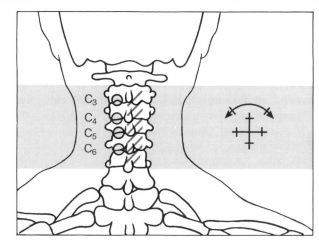

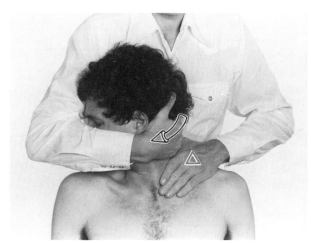

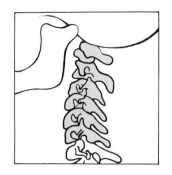

## Mobilization with Impulse (Thrust): Rotation Side-Bending Restriction

### Indication (Fig. a)

*Zone of irritation:* C2, C3, C4, C5, C6, C7, T1, T2, T3.

*Motion testing:* Segmental or regional rotation or sidebending restriction with hard endfeel.

*Pain:* Localized; occasional pseudoradicular radiation to the arms and the area between the scapulae.

### Positioning

- The patient is seated and the operator stands at the patient's side.
- The operator fixates with one hand the patient's head in the temporal region. The middle and index fingers of the other hand are placed over the articular pillar of the vertebra above the segment that is to be mobilized (Fig. **b**).
- Passive side-bending and rotation are introduced, bringing the spinal segment to the pathologic barrier. Slight traction is also applied (Fig. **c**).

### Treatment Procedure

- The impulse is effected through the articular pillar, the force being directed antero-superiorly along the planes of the facets (Fig. **d**).

*Note:* The fixating hand should not provide additional impulse forces.

### Remarks

This is an excellent technique for the anxious or non-relaxed patient.

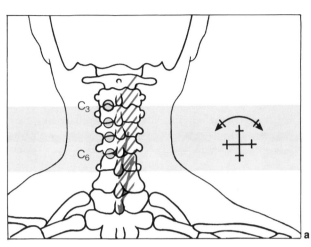

a

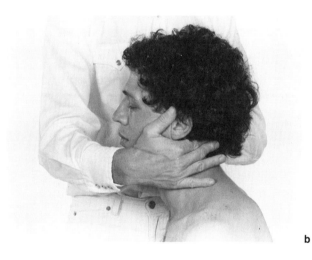

b

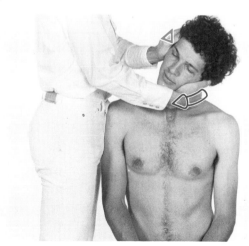

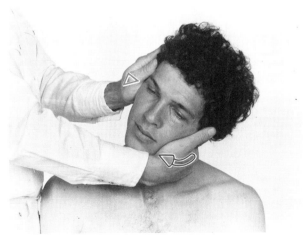

c

# C2 to T3

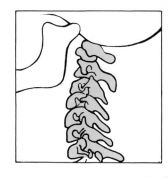

## NMT 1 and Self-Mobilization: Rotation Restriction

### Indication (Fig. a)

*Zone of irritation:* C2, C3, C4, C5, C6, C7, T1, T2, T3.

*Motion testing:* Segmental or regional rotation and side-bending restriction with hard endfeel.

*Pain:* Chronic in the neck region radiating to the shoulders and arms, occasionally radiating to the occiput and the region between the shoulder blades.

*Muscle testing:* Shortening of the descending portion of the trapezius and levator scapulae muscles; occasional weakening of the muscles that hold the shoulder blade in place.

### Positioning

- The patient is seated.
- The articular processes of the vertebra below the restricted spinal segment are fixated by the index and middle fingers of one hand with the remainder of the hand lying flat over the lower cervical spine.
- The spinal segments above the involved segment are inclined (C0–C1) and flexed (C2–T2) until the involved segment is localized (Fig. **b**).
- Self-mobilization: The lower vertebra of the restricted spinal segment is fixated by the operator's fifth metacarpal and small finger on that side to which mobilization is to take place. The cervical spinal segments above the restricted segment are inclined or flexed, localizing the involved segment (Fig. **c**).

*Note:* If pain becomes manifest while localizing the restricted spinal segment, the segments C0 to C3 should be examined first and, if indicated, treated.

### Treatment Procedure

- Active rotation mobilization is performed with the patient looking in the same direction as his rotation.

### Remarks

Self-mobilization techniques are well suited for patients who have recurrent somatic dysfunctions and pain that may be due to their gross movements and posture during work, i.e., typists ("stereotype posture").

Almost always mobilization must be performed before the trapezius muscle can be stretched.

If pain becomes manifest during mobilization, the following cause may be responsible:

- Undue pressure over the zone of irritation.

If short-term improvement is followed by significant worsening, post-traumatic instability should be considered.

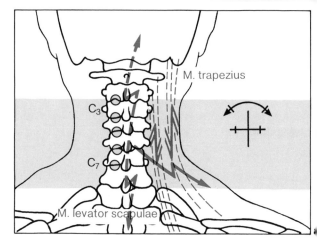

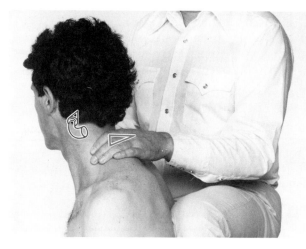

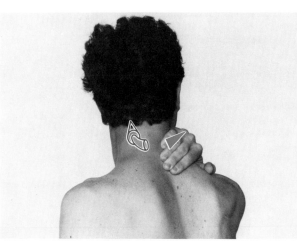

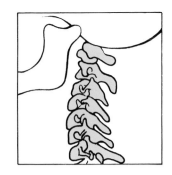

## NMT 2: Rotation Restriction

### Indication (Fig. a)

*Zone of irritation:* C3, C4, C5, C6, C7, T1, T2, T3.
*Motion testing:* Segmental rotation restriction with soft endfeel.
*Pain:* Chronic in neck region; occasionally radiating to the arms.
*Muscle testing:* Shortening of the descending portion of the trapezius and levator scapulae muscles; weakening of the medial aspects of those muscles that hold the shoulder blade in place and the erector spinae muscles in the thoracic region.

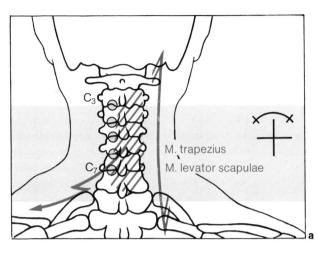

### Positioning

– Patient is seated.
– The cervical spine is in the anatomic position or the present neutral position.
– The lower vertebra of the restricted spinal segment is softly fixated by thumb and index finger through the articular pillars.
– The head and upper cervical area are embraced. The fifth metacarpal and small finger are placed over the articular processes of the vertebra above the incriminated spinal segment (Fig.**b**).
– The restricted spinal segment is carried to its pathologic barrier.

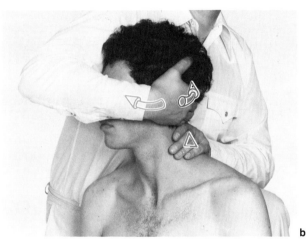

### Treatment Procedure:

– Isometric muscle contraction away from the pathologic barrier with the patient's gaze in the direction of rotation (Fig. **b**).
– Passive mobilization, along with axial traction, is introduced during the postisometric relaxation phase in order to move beyond the pathologic barrier.

### Remarks

The path gained with each individual mobilization step is rather small.
If several segments are restricted at once, one should start with the segment that exhibits the most pronounced zone of irritation.
If radicular pain appears during mobilization, the procedure should be terminated at once and be replaced by other techniques.
One may resort to:
– Mobilization without impulse
– NMT 1
– Possibly mobilization with impulse in selected cases.
If excessive pressure is applied to the zone of irritation, significant localized pain may appear.

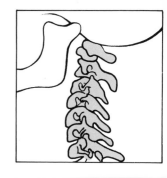

## NMT 2 and NMT 3: Side-Bending Restriction

### Indication (Fig. a)

*Zone of irritation:* C2, C3, C4, C5, C6, C7, T1, T2, T3.

*Motion testing:* Segmental sidebending restriction with soft endfeel.

*Pain:* Localized or radiating to the arms.

*Muscle testing:* Shortening of the descending portions of the trapezius and levator scapulae muscles. Weakening of the medial aspects of those muscles that hold the shoulder blade in place.

*Autonomic symptoms:* Position-dependent nonsystematic vertigo. Numbness of the arms during sleep.

*Note:* When dealing with an isolated side-bending restriction, one should think of spondylogenic changes affecting the lateral portions of the vertebral body borders (uncal region). Due to the close proximity to the vertebral artery and the spinal nerve, a local mechanical factor may often be involved.

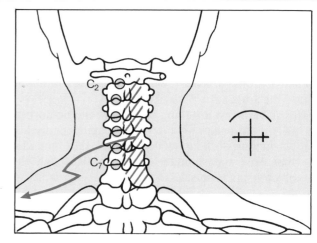

### Positioning

- Patient is seated.
- The patient's cervical spine is brought to its anatomic position or present neutral position.
- The lower of the two vertebrae of the restricted spinal segment is fixated by the operator placing his thumb and index finger over the articular pillars.
- The operator embraces the patient's head and upper cervical spine, while the fifth metacarpal and small finger are placed over the articular pillar of the vertebra directly above the incriminated spinal segment (Fig. **b**).
- The restricted spinal segment is carried to its pathologic barrier.

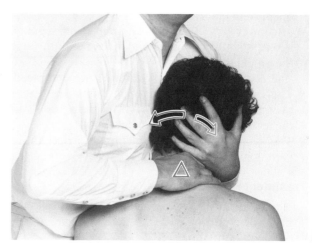

### Treatment Procedure

- NMT 2: isometric contraction away from the pathologic barrier.
- Passive side-bending movement is introduced during the postisometric relaxation phase. Movement is effected through the operator's chest and upper hand. Slight traction is also applied (Fig. **b**).
- NMT 3: isometric contraction toward the pathologic motion barrier.
  Passive side-bending movement is then introduced during the relaxation phase.

### Remarks

If vertigo becomes manifest during treatment, the procedure should be terminated at once and replaced by one of the following, less forceful, techniques.
- Traction
- Mobilization with and without impulse
- NMT 1

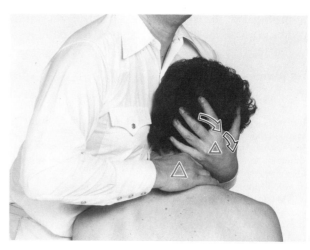

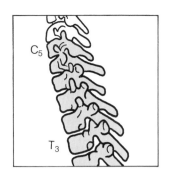

## Mobilization with Impulse (Thrust): Rotation and Side-Bending Restriction

### Indications (Fig. a)

*Zone of irritation:* C5, C6, C7, T1, T2, T3, T4.

*Motion testing:* Segmental motion restriction with hard endfeel.

*Pain:* Cervical and thoracic regions; occasionally radiating to the arms and hands and the region between the scapulae.

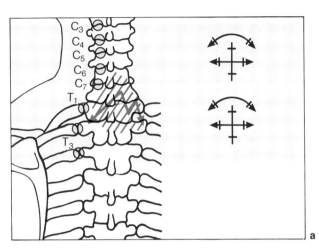

### Positioning

- The patient is sitting somewhat slouched and with the cervical spine flexed.
- The operator standing behind the patient places his thumb laterally over the spinous process of the vertebra above the spinal segment that is to be mobilized. In no case should the lateral triangle of the neck be touched with the other fingers.
- The other arm then cradles the patient's head, and the hypothenar is placed over the articular pillar of the vertebra above the spinal segment that is to be mobilized (Fig. **b**).
- Through his cradling arm, the operator introduces passive rotation, bringing the spinal segment to its pathologic barrier.

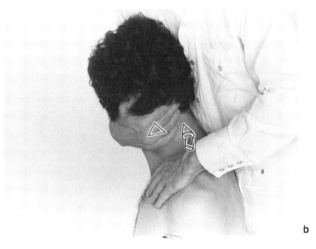

### Treatment Procedure

- During the exhalation phase, the impulse is effected through the operator's thumb against the spinous process (Figs. **b, c**).

### Remarks

Under no circumstances must the lateral triangle of the neck be compressed.

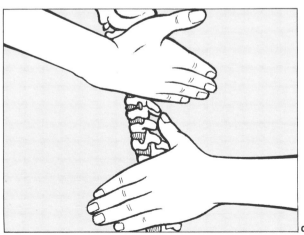

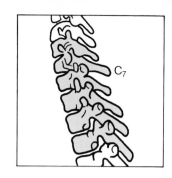

## NMT 1, Self-Mobilization, Mobilization without Impulse: Extension Restriction

### Indication (Fig. a)

*Zone of irritation:* C6, C7, T1, T2, T3, T4.
*Motion testing:* Segmental extension restriction with hard or soft endfeel.
*Pain:* Localized.
*Muscle testing:* Shortening of the levator scapulae muscle.

### Positioning

– Patient is supine with his legs flexed.
– The vertebra below the involved spinal segment is fixated at the spinous process by the operator's hand or a sandbag (Figs. **b**, **c**).
– The upper cervical spine is supported by requesting the patient to cross his hands behind his neck.

### Treatment Procedure

– NMT 1, self-mobilization: active extension mobilization during the inhalation phase (Fig. **b**).
– Mobilization without impulse: passive mobilization utilizing gravity force. The operator may provide additional support by pressing against the patient's elbows (Fig. **c**).

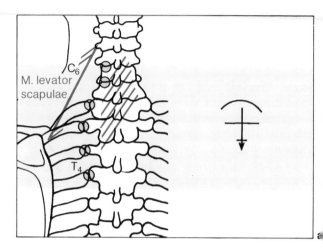

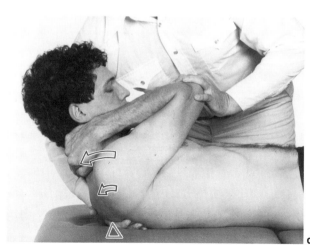

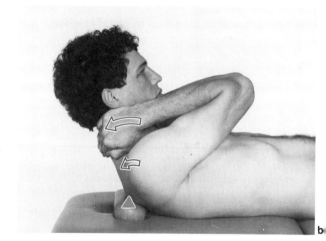

# C6 to T4

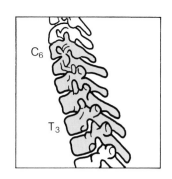

## Mobilization with Impulse (Thrust): Rotation Restriction

### Indication (Fig. a)

*Zone of irritation:* C6, C7, T1, T2, T3, T4.
*Motion testing:* Segmental motion restriction with hard endfeel.
*Pain:* Cervical and thoracic regions; radiating into the arms and the area between the scapulae.

### Positioning

- The patient is seated, clasping his hands behind his neck without pulling it forward, however.
- Standing at the patient's side, the operator takes hold of the patient's arms from inferior (Fig. **b**).
- He places the thumb of the other hand laterally on the spinous process of the vertebra below the spinal segment that is to be mobilized.
- Through the patient's arms, he introduces passive rotation, bringing the segment to the pathologic barrier.
- The thoracic kyphosis is exaggerated (introduce flexion).

### Treatment Procedure

- During exhalation, the impulse is directed toward the spinous process (Fig. **c**).

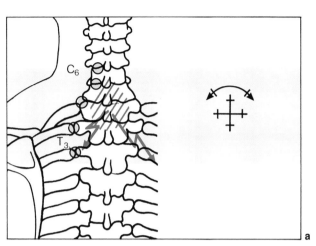

a

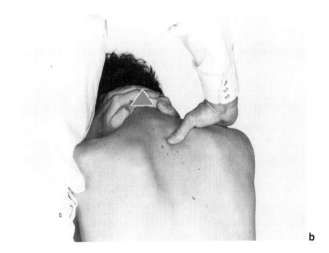

b

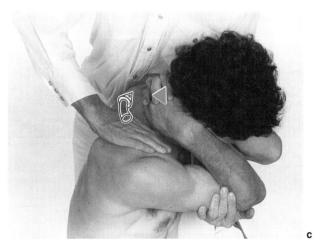

c

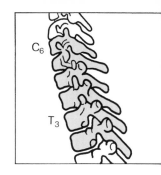

## Mobilization with Impulse (Thrust): Rotation, Side-Bending Restriction in Extension

### Indication (Fig. a)

*Zone of irritation:* C6, C7, T1, T2, T3, T4.
*Motion testing:* Segmental or regional motion restriction with hard endfeel.
*Pain:* Cervical and thoracic areas; radiating into the arms and the regions between the scapulae.

### Positioning

- The patient is prone with the thoracic and cervical spine slightly flexed.
- The operator stands at the patient's side holding the head with both hands, then passively side-bends and rotates it to the side on which he stands (Fig. **b**).
- Change of hands: While one hand is placed broadly over the patient's shoulder, the other hand remains in contact with the patient's head. Thus, the arms are now crossed, with the forearms being parallel to each other (Fig. **c**).

### Treatment Procedure

- During exhalation a lateral-inferior impulse is effected through the hand that rests on the patient's shoulder (Fig. **c**).

*Note:* Specific mobilization is possible as long as the thumb of the hand providing the impulse is placed laterally over the spinous process of the vertebra inferior to the spinal segment that is to be mobilized (Fig. **d**).
It may be helpful to lower the head piece of the treatment table, since one can introduce greater flexion to the cervicothoracic junction more easily.

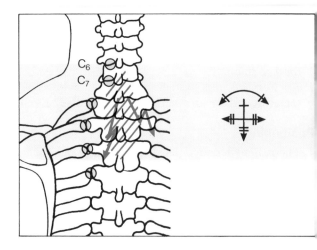

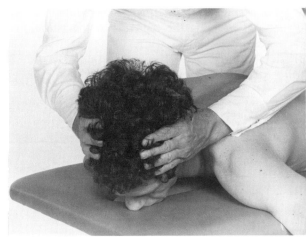

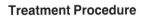

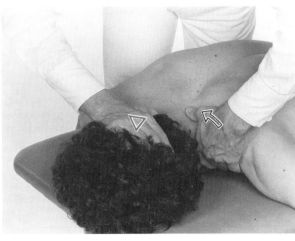

d

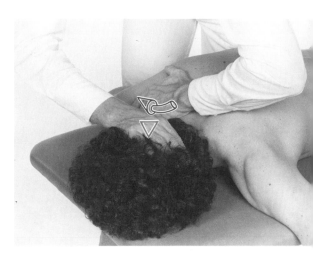

## Mobilization without Impulse: Rotation Restriction

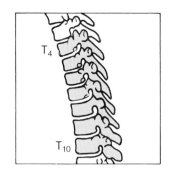

### Indication (Fig. a)

*Zone of irritation:* T3, T4, T5, T6, T7, T8, T9, T10.
*Motion testing:* Segmental rotation restriction with hard or soft endfeel.
*Pain:* Localized or segmental; radiating toward the sternum.

### Positioning

- The patient is sitting with his arms crossed in front of his chest and the hands resting on the shoulder.
- The operator placing his one arm anteriorly around the patient rests the hand on the shoulder.
- The restricted segment is rotated to its pathologic barrier.
- The operator places his other hand over the transverse process of the superior joint partner (vertebra) of the restricted spinal segment (Fig. **b**).

### Treatment Procedure

- The operator steadily increases the pressure over the spinous process of the inferior vertebra of the restricted spinal segment, thereby effecting passive mobilization. Careful rotation is also introduced to the entire thoracic spine (Fig.**b**).

### Remarks

This technique can be applied only if one deals with isolated, well-localized restriction findings.
One should not apply this technique if there are other concomitant problems in:
- The sacroiliac joints
- The lumbar spine
- Complex presentations in the thoracic spine

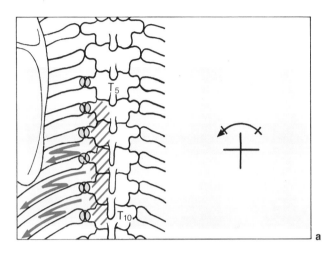

a

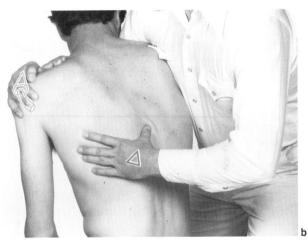

b

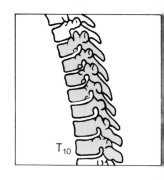

## Mobilization without Impulse and NMT 2: Extension Restriction

### Indication (Fig. a)

*Zone of irritation:* T3, T4, T5, T6, T7, T8, T9, T10.

*Motion testing:* Segmental or regional extension restriction with possible side-bending restriction. Rather hard endfeel.

*Pain:* Acute or chronic. May be related to respiratory movement. Pain radiates on a segmental level toward the sternum or may be localized.

*Muscle testing:* Weakening of the thoracic portion of the erector spinae muscle and those muscles holding the shoulder blade in place medially. The levator scapulae muscle is often shortened.

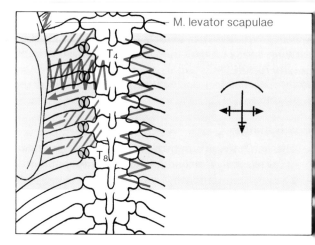

M. levator scapulae

### Positioning

- The patient is supine with his legs flexed and arms crossed in front of the chest.
- The operator rotates the patient passively toward himself and fixates the inferior vertebra of the involved segment with his thenar eminence and flexed middle finger over the transverse processes (Fig. **b**).

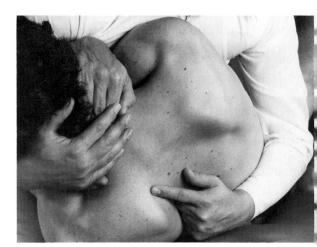

## Mobilization without Impulse and NMT 2: Extension Restriction (cont'd.)

### Treatment Procedure

– Mobilization without impulse: The patient is rotated onto his back. During mobilization, the gravity force is utilized while additional force is applied to patient's elbows to increase extension (Fig. **c**).

– NMT 2: The incriminated spinal segment is extended until the pathologic barrier is engaged. The muscles responsible for flexion are contracted isometrically to optimum.

– During the postisometric relaxation phase, the spinal segment is passively mobilized in the direction of extension beyond the motion barrier (Fig. **d**).

*Note:* The isometric contraction is during the inhalation phase, whereas mobilization is during the inhalation phase.

### Remarks

The inferior vertebra can also be fixated with a sandbag.

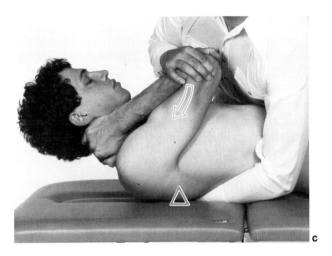

c

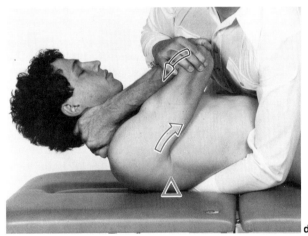

d

## Mobilization without Impulse and NMT 2: Rotation Restriction

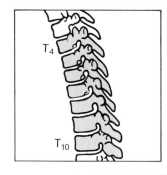

### Indication (Fig. a)

*Zone of irritation:* T3, T4, T5, T6, T7, T8, T9, T10.
*Motion testing:* Segmental rotation restriction with hard endfeel.
*Pain:* Acute or chronic, segmental; localized or radiating toward the sternum.
*Muscle testing:* Shortening of the semispinalis, multifidi and rotatores muscles.

### Positioning

– Patient is in the side-lying position.
– Exact localization and preparation is achieved in two steps. In the first step the vertebrae below the involved spinal segment are rotated until the restricted segment is reached and all the slack is taken up. In the second step, the vertebrae above the incriminated segment are rotated down to the involved segment.
– The operator fixates the superior vertebra of the involved segment with his fingertips. The point of fixation is on the spinous process, on the side away from the table.
– The operator places the fingertips of the opposite hand over the side of the spinous process that points toward the table (Fig. **b**).
– The spinal segment is carried to its pathologic barrier.

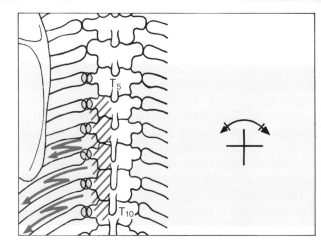

### Treatment Procedure

– *Mobilization without impulse:* Passive rotation is introduced by mobilization applying direct traction to the spinous process of the inferior vertebra. In addition, the inferior vertebrae are also rotated at the same thime (Fig. **b**).
– *NMT 2:* Isometric rotation away from the motion barrier (inhalation).
– During the postisometric relaxation phase, the segment is mobilized beyond its pathologic barrier (exhalation) (Fig. **c**).

### Remarks

The operator should avoid leaning on the patient.

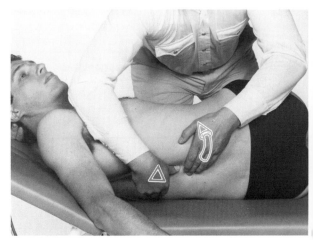

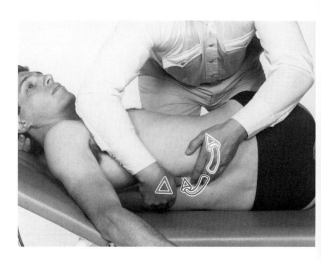

## Mobilization with Impulse (Thrust): Flexion Restriction

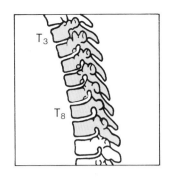

### Indication (Fig. a)

*Zone of irritation:* T3, T4, T5, T6, T7, T8, T9, T10.
*Motion testing:* Segmental or regional restriction with hard endfeel.
*Pain:* Midthoracic spine; beltlike radiation.

### Positioning

– Patient is prone.
– The involved spinal segment or area is exactly localized and engaged by introducing flexion to the thoracic spine (exaggerated kyphosis).
– The operator places his hands broadly over both transverse processes (thenar eminence) and the respective ribs (the palm of the hand and hypothenar).
– The operator's forearms are nearly tangential to the involved portion of the spine (Fig. **b**).

### Treatment Procedure

– Passive mobilization is effected through both hands, providing a superiorly and slightly anteriorly directed impulse force (Fig. **c**).

### Remarks

The impulse receives an additional rotation component if the operator slides his hand over the next adjoining segment.

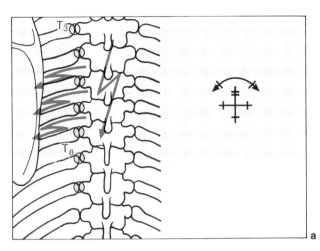

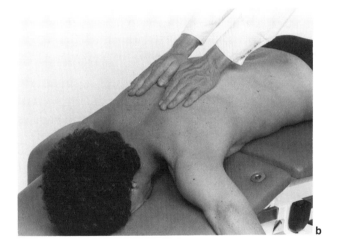

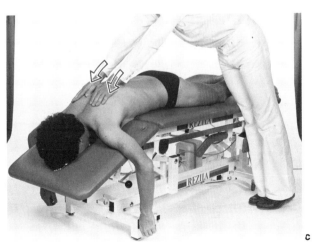

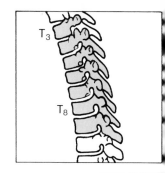

## Mobilization with Impulse (Thrust): Extension-Rotation Restriction

### Indication (Fig. a)

*Zone of irritation:* T3, T4, T5, T6, T7, T8, T9, T10.
*Motion testing:* Segmental restriction with hard end-feel.
*Pain:* Thoracic spine.

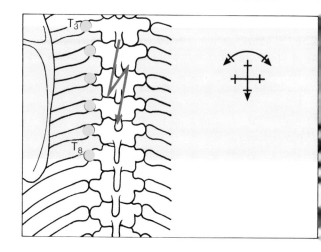

### Positioning

- The patient is supine with his hands clasped behind his neck.
- The operator rotates the patient passively toward him, holding with one hand the patient's neck and head in order to monitor flexion in the cervicothoracic junction (Fig. **b**).
- The thumb and index finger of the other hand are straight while the fingers III to V are flexed.
- The thenar eminence of that hand is placed over the transverse process of the vertebra inferior to the spinal segment that is to be mobilized. The bent middle finger is placed over the transverse process of the vertebra above the spinal segment that is to be mobilized (Fig. **c**).
- The patient is then rotated back to the supine position.

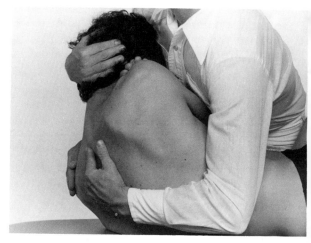

### Treatment Procedure

- During exhalation, the operator effects an impulse through the patient's arms (Fig. **d**).
- Due to the way the fingers are placed, the impulse has a rotational extension effect.

### Remarks

As an alternative to having the patient's hands clasped behind his neck, one may instruct the patient to cross the arms over his chest.

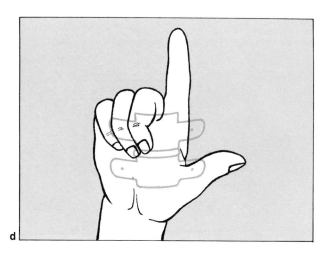

d

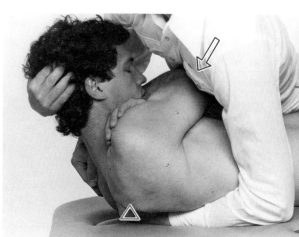

## Mobilization with Impulse (Thrust): Rotation Restriction

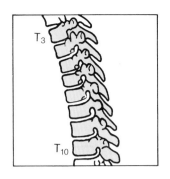

### Indication (Fig. a)

*Zone of irritation:* T3, T4, T5, T6, T7, T8, T9, T10.
*Motion testing:* Segmental or regional restriction with hard endfeel.
*Pain:* Midthoracic spine; the pain may radiate in a beltlike manner.

### Positioning

- Patient is prone.
- The spinal segment that is to be mobilized is localized by introducing flexion to the thoracic spine.
- The operator stands at the patient's side. The pisiform bone of one hand is placed over the transverse process of the vertebra below the restricted spinal segment while the pisiform bone of the other hand is placed over the transverse process of the vertebra above the restricted spinal segment.
- The arms are crossed, with the forearms forming an angle of 45° against the vertebral column (Fig. **b**).
- During exhalation, pressure is applied to the transverse processes guiding the spinal segment to its pathologic barrier.

### Treatment Procedure

- At the end of exhalation, both hands introduce an impulse in the anterior direction (Fig. **b**).

### Remarks

Please note:
- The pisiform bone should not make contact with the ribs, since otherwise it may exacerbate the patient's symptoms.

In cases in which the pain becomes worse with the application of anterior pressure on the transverse processes, the treatment procedure must be discontinued.

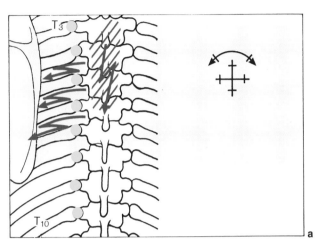

a

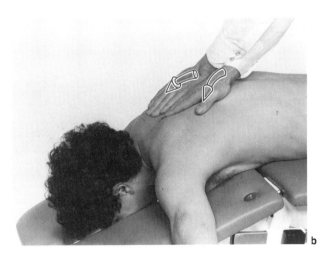

b

## Mobilization with Impulse (Thrust): Rotation Restriction

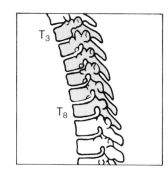

### Indication (Fig. a)

*Zone of irritation:* T3, T4, T5, T6, T7, T8, T9, T10.
*Motion testing:* Segmental restriction with hard end-feel.
*Pain:* In the thoracic area, radiating in a beltlike manner.

### Positioning

- The patient is prone with flexion being introduced to the thoracic spine until the incriminated segment is localized and engaged.
- The operator crosses his hands in such a manner that the anatomic snuffbox of the left hand touches the right ulnar styloid process. The ulnar border of the left hand becomes the guiding hand, which is placed along the right side of the spinous processes (Fig. **b**). The fingers point in the superior direction.
- The pisiform bone of the right hand is placed over the transverse process of the thoracic vertebra above on the opposite side (Figs. **c, d**).

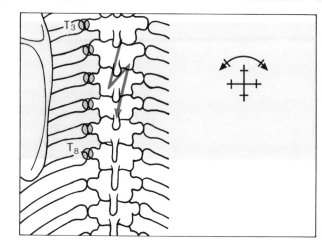

### Treatment Procedure

- The impulse is effected through the pisiform bone, as the operator slightly flexes his elbows.
- The impulse in this technique is also effected at the moment in which the patient has exhaled maximally (Figs. **c, d**).

### Remarks

This technique should not be utilized in situations in which there is anterior displacement of a spinal segment. Also, one should be careful when utilizing the technique on elderly patients.

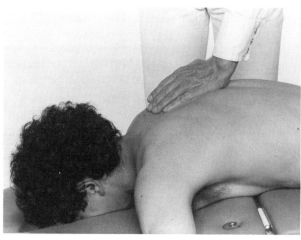

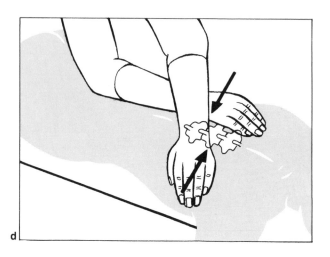

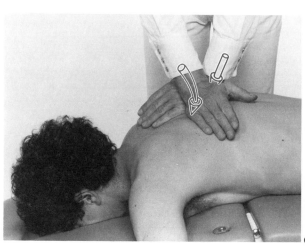

# T8 to T12

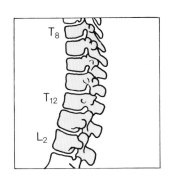

## Mobilization with Impulse (Thrust): Rotation Restriction

### Indication (Fig. a)

*Zone of irritation:* T8, T9, T10, T11, T12.
*Motion testing:* Segmental restriction with hard end-feel.
*Pain:* Localized with occasional associated flank pain.

### Positioning

– Patient is in the side-lying position close to the edge of examination table.
– The operator fixates with one hand the patient's pelvis while with the other hand he grasps the patient's forearm and brings the shoulder close to the table toward him. The opposite shoulder (the one away from the table) is rotated away, introducing rotation into the thoracic spine.
– The thoracic spine is rotated to the pathologic barrier of the spinal segment that is to be mobilized.
– The patient is fixated in this position by the operator either stabilizing the patient's shoulder or placing his elbow against the patient's axilla.
– One is now ready to localize the involved spinal segment from inferior. The operator places his hand over the patient's pelvis, introducing passive flexion to the hip through the upper leg (the leg away from the table) thereby introducing flexion to the lumbar spine as well. The foot of the upper leg is then placed against the poplitea of the lower leg. The operator places his knee against the lateral aspect of the poplitea of the patient's flexed leg in order to control further movement.
– The operator (upper arm) fixates the vertebra above the spinal segment that is to be mobilized. The point of fixation is through the spinous process, in particular the side that points away from the table.
– The fingertips of the other hand (lower arm) are placed over the spinous process of the vertebra below the spinal segment that is to mobilized. Here, contact is made with the side of the spinous process that is toward the table. The forearm rests on the pelvis (Fig. **b**).

### Treatment Procedure

– Through the hand of the lower arm, an anteroinferior impulse is effected against the spinous process (Fig. **c**).

### Remarks

It is important to have exact localization and good fixation.
If the patient reports pain with positioning, it is most likely due to insufficient lumbar spine flexion.

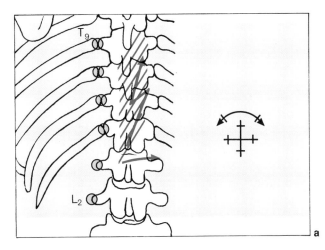

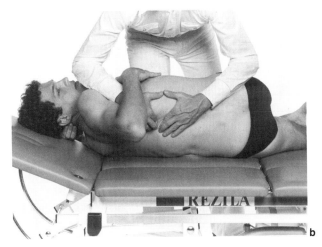

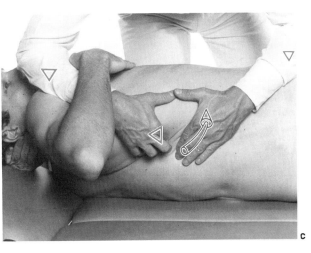

## Mobilization with Impulse (Thrust): Rotation Restriction

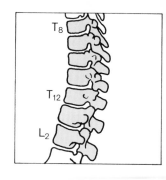

### Indication (Fig. a)

*Zone of irritation:* T8, T9, T10, T11, T12.
*Motion testing:* Regional motion restriction with hard endfeel.
*Pain:* Localized or radiating to the flanks.

### Positioning

– The patient is sitting astride the examination table with his hands crossed over his chest.
– The operator, standing behind the patient, reaches around the patient in front with one arm and introduces in that way passive rotation and simultaneous slight flexion to the thoracic spinal areas.
– The pisiform bone of the other hand is placed over the transverse process of the vertebra above the involved spinal segment (Figs. **b, c**).
– Rotation is continued until the restricted segment is engaged at its pathologic barrier.

### Treatment Procedure

During exhalation, a rotatory impulse is effected against the transverse process and at an angle corresponding to that of the inclination of the joint surfaces (Fig. **c**).

### Remarks

Modification: If the pisiform bone is placed over the angle of the rib, the rib will be mobilized, which in turn will mobilize the corresponding thoracic segment indirectly.

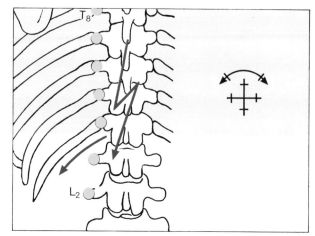

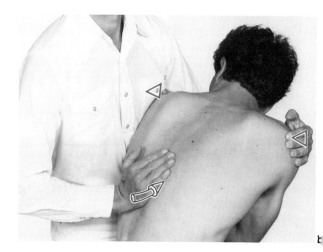

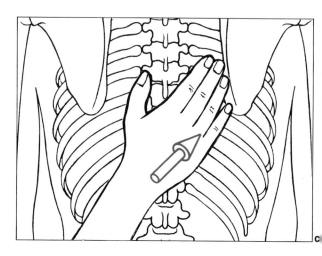

# T10 to Sacrum

## Mobilization without Impulse: Rotation Restriction

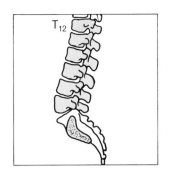

### Indication (Fig. a)

*Zone of irritation:* T10, T11, T12, L1, L2, L3, L4, L5, S1.

*Motion testing:* Segmental rotation and side-bending motion restriction with rather hard endfeel.

*Pain:* Localized and chronic.

*Muscle testing:* The lumbar portion of the erector spinae muscle and the quadratus lumborum muscle are shortened.

### Positioning

– The patient is sitting with his arms crossed in front and hands resting on his shoulders.
– The vertebrae above the restricted segment are flexed and rotated in order to bring the restricted segment to its pathologic barrier (Fig. **b**).
– Operator places his thumb over the spinous process of the vertebra below the restricted spinal segment.

### Treatment Procedure

Mobilization is effected by passively rotating the shoulder girdle and thoracic spine (Fig. **b**).

### Remarks

This is a rather nonspecific mobilization technique.

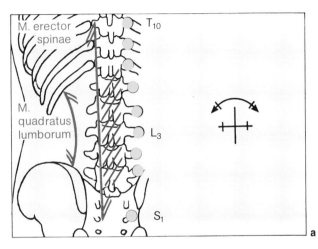

a

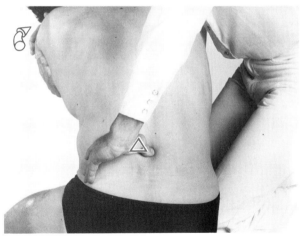

b

# T12 to Sacrum

## Mobilization without Impulse and NMT 2: Rotation Restriction

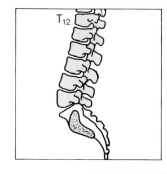

### Indication (Fig. a)

*Zone of irritation:* T12, L1, L2, L3, L4, L5, S.

*Motion testing:* Segmental rotation and side-bending motion restriction with hard or soft endfeel.

*Remarks:* If the endfeel is hard, one should employ mobilization techniques without impulse, whereas in the event of soft endfeel NMT 2 should be utilized.

*Pain:* Chronic or acute; localized.

*Muscle testing:* The piriformis and erector spinae muscles (lumbar portion) are shortened; the quadratus lumborum muscle may be shortened in some instances.

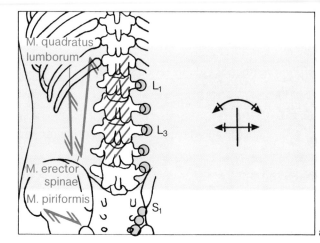

### Positioning

– Patient is in the side lying position.
– First the vertebrae below, then the vertebrae above the restricted segment are rotated in order to exactly localize the restricted segment.
– The operator fixates the superior vertebra of the restricted segment by placing his fingertips over the spinous process, the portion that is pointing away from the table.
– The operator then places his fingertips of the other hand over the spinous process of the inferior vertebra of the restricted segment. Point of fixation is the side close to the table (Fig. **b**).
– The spinal segment is subsequently carried to its pathologic barrier.

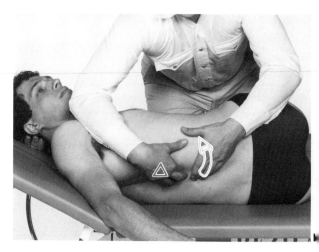

### Treatment Procedure

– *Mobilization without impulse:* The operator introduces direct traction to the inferior spinous process, thereby effecting passive rotation mobilization. The inferior vertebrae are simultaneously rotated while traction is imployed (Fig. **b**).
– *NMT 2:* Isometric rotation away from the restrictive barrier (during inspiration). During the postisometric relaxation phase, mobilization carries the segment beyond the pathologic barrier (during exhalation) (Fig. **c**).

### Remarks

Since the zone of irritation is in close proximity to the point of fixation, one should place his hands rather broadly over that area. Rotation of the vetebrae below the restricted spinal segment can cause problems, especially if the sacroiliac joint is diseased as well. This, however, must be differentiated from a shortened piriformis muscle.

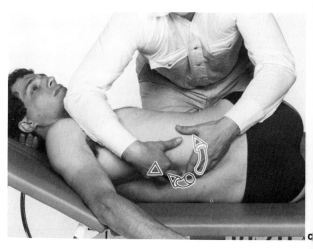

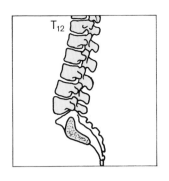

## Self-Mobilization and NMT 1: Rotation Restriction

### Indication (Fig. a)

*Zone of irritation:* T10, T11, T12, L1, L2, L3, L4, L5, S.

*Motion testing:* Segmental rotation and side-bending motion restriction. Abrupt or soft endfeel during passive motion testing.

*Pain:* Chronic and localized.

*Muscle testing:* The erector spinae muscle is shortened in the lumbar area. The quadratus lumborum muscle may sometimes be shortened as well.

### Positioning

- Patient is in side-lying position. The pelvis is stabilized by flexing the upper leg. Rotation is introduced from superior until the restricted segment is localized.
- The operator fixates the inferior vertebra of the restricted spinal segment by placing his fingertips over the spinous process. The forearm rests on the pelvic crest and the greater trochanter, providing further stabilization (Fig. b).

### Treatment Procedure

- NMT 1 (Fig. b) and self-mobilization (Fig. c). The restricted segment it carried to its pathologic barrier.
- Active rotation mobilization beyond the pathologic barrier is effected.
- The patient's gaze should be in the same direction as rotation.

### Remarks

When positioning the patient, one should make sure that the lumbar spine is in its neutral position or slightly flexed. There should be no lumbar extension.

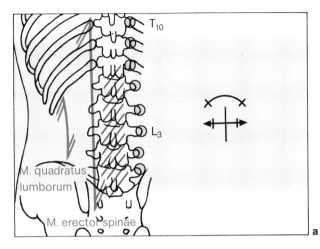

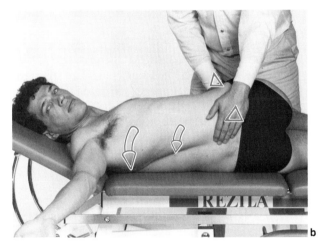

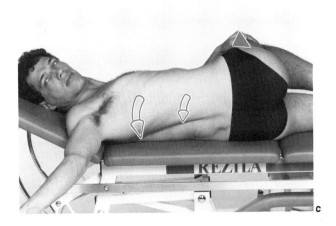

# L1 to L5

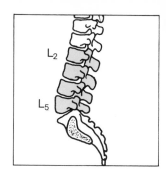

## Mobilization with Impulse (Thrust): Rotation Restriction

### Indication (Fig. a)

*Zone of irritation:* L1, L2, L3, L4, L5.

*Motion testing:* Regional motion restriction with hard endfeel.

*Pain:* Localized or radiating to the legs and the buttock region.

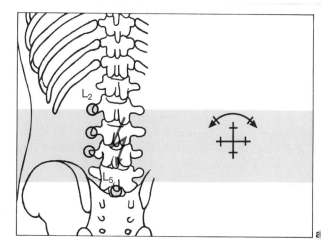

### Positioning

- The patient is in the side-lying position, close to the edge of the examination table. The operator fixates the patient's pelvis with one hand.
- With the other hand, he grasps the patient's lower arm, drawing the shoulder (the one close to the table) toward him.
- The shoulder pointing away from the table is rotated, whereby rotation to the thoracic spine is introduced.

  The thoracic and lumbar spines are rotated until the pathologic barrier of the incriminated spinal segment is localized and engaged. The operator then fixates the patient in this position either through the patient's shoulder or by placing his elbow against the patient's axilla.
- The patient is then asked to move his eyes in the same direction as rotation, allowing reflexive relaxation of the back musculature.
- The resticted spinal segments can now be localized from inferior in the following manner: With the hand over the patient's pelvis, the operator introduces passive flexion to the hip, thereby effecting flexion in the lumbar spine. The patient's foot comes to rest against the poplitea of the lower leg (the leg near the table).
- The operator places his knee over the lateral aspect of the poplitea of the patient's flexed leg for monitoring. The lumbar spine and pelvis are rotated so that the anterior iliac spine comes to rest on the examination table. To achieve this, one may sometimes have to reverse some of the originally established thoracic and lumbar spine rotation.

## Mobilization with Impulse (Thrust): Rotation Restriction (cont'd.)

– The mobilizing hand is now placed flat over the sacrum and the spinous process of L5. The forearm rests on the buttock. The operator shifts his point of gravity superiorly, which introduces further tension. The fixating knee also moves superiorly at the same time. With the spine engaged and positioned in this manner, the impulse is introduced and directed toward the sacrum and L5, following an anteroinferior direction (Figs. **b, c**)

### Treatment Procedure

– The spinal segment is carried to its pathologic barrier.
– The impulse is in an anterior direction (rotation); for the spinal segment L5–S1, it is directed inferiorly.

### Remarks

One should note:
– The patient should be totally relaxed.
– The impulse should be applied during exhalation.
– If the patient has arthrosis of the hip (coxarthrosis) the patient cannot be stabilized by flexing his upper leg. Since it is important, however, to have good stabilization, the operator places his forearm against the patient's pelvis as firmly as possible.

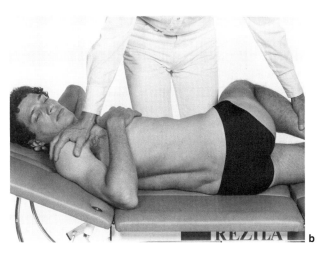
b

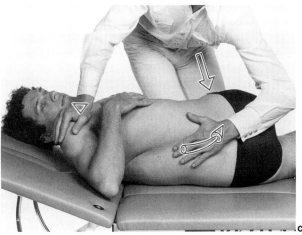
c

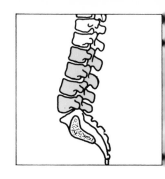

## Mobilization with Impulse (Thrust): Rotation Restriction

### Indication (Fig. a)

*Zone of irritation:* L1, L2, L3, L4, L5.

*Motion testing:* Segmental rotation motion restriction with hard endfeel.

*Pain:* Localized or radiating to the legs and the buttock region.

### Positioning

– Patient is in the sidelying position close to the edge of the table.

– The operator fixates with one hand the patient's pelvis while with the other he reaches around the patient's lower arm, pulling the shoulder that is close to the table toward him.

– The shoulder pointing away from the table is rotated away from the operator, introducing rotation to the thoracic spine.

– Rotation in the thoracic and lumbar spine is carried to its barrier, localizing exactly the restricted spinal segment.

– The operator fixates the patient in this position either through the patient's shoulder or by placing his elbow at the patient's axilla.

– The patient follows with his eyes the direction of rotation, allowing reflexive relaxation of the back musculature.

– One is now able to localize the restrictive segment from inferiorly:
With his fixating hand, the operator introduces passive flexion to the hip, thereby effecting flexion in the lumbar spine. The patient's foot comes to rest against the poplitea of the lower leg.

– The operator places his knee over the lateral aspect of the poplitea of the patient's flexed leg for further monitoring. The lumbar spine and pelvis are rotated so that the anterior iliac spine comes to rest on the examination table. One may sometimes have to reverse the originally established thoracic and lumbar spine rotation.

– The operator places the pisiform bone of his inferior hand over the spinous process of the vertebra below the restricted segment. Specific localization at the spinous process is at the side away from the table (Figs. **b, c**).

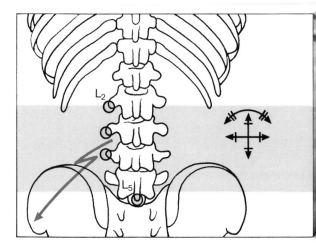

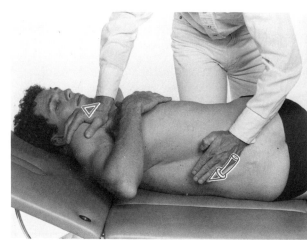

## Mobilization with Impulse (Thrust): Rotation Restriction (cont'd.)

### Treatment Procedure

- The spinal segment is carried to its pathologic barrier.
- During exhalation, a rotatory impulse force is effected through the pisiform bone against the spinous process (toward the examination table) (Fig. **c**).

### Remarks

If the patient has painful arthrosis of the hip (coxarthrosis), one should not stabilize the patient by flexing the upper leg. Since stabilization is important, however, the operator should place his forearm against the patient's pelvis as securely as the situation allows.

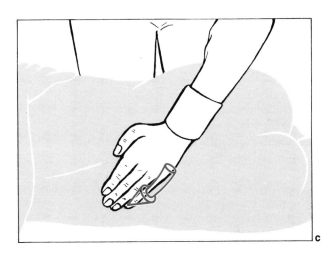

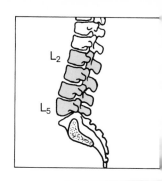

## Mobilization with Impulse (Thrust): Rotation and Flexion Restriction

### Indication (Fig. a)

*Zone of irritation:* L1, L2, L3, L4, L5.
*Motion testing:* Segmental motion restriction with hard endfeel.
*Pain:* Local or radiation to the gluteal region or legs.

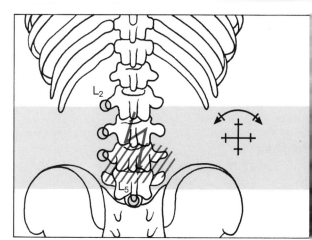

### Positioning

- Patient is in the side-lying position close to the edge of the table.
- The operator fixates with one hand the patient's pelvis while with the other he reaches around the patient's lower arm, pulling the shoulder that is close to the table toward him.
- The shoulder pointing away from the table is rotated away from the operator, introducing rotation to the thoracic spine.
- Rotation in the thoracic and lumbar spine is carried to its barrier, localizing and engaging the restricted spinal segment.
- The operator fixates the patient in this position either through the patient's shoulder or by placing his elbow at the patient's axilla.
- The patient follows with his eyes the direction of rotation, allowing reflexive relaxation of the back musculature.
- One is now able to localize and engage the restrictive segment from inferiorly. With his fixating hand, the operator introduces passive flexion to the hip, thereby effecting flexion in the lumbar spine. The patient's foot comes to rest against the poplitea of the lower leg.
- The operator places his knee over the lateral aspect of the poplitea of the patient's flexed leg for further monitoring. The lumbar spine and pelvis are rotated so that the anterior iliac spine comes to rest on the examination table. One may sometimes have to reverse the originally established thoracic and lumbar spine rotation.

## Mobilization with Impulse (Thrust): Rotation and Flexion Restriction (cont'd.)

– The operator fixates with the fingertips of his upper hand the spinous process of the vertebra above the segment that is to be mobilized. The localization at the spinous process is on the side away from the table.

– The fingertips of the other hand are placed over the spinous process of the vertebra below the spinal segment that is to be mobilized. Localization at the spinous process, here, is at the side facing the table. The forearm rests on the patient's pelvis.

### Treatment Procedure

– The spinal segment is carried to its pathologic barrier.

– During exhalation, the impulse is effected through the lower hand against the spinous process in the lateral and inferior direction, according to the spatial arrangement of the joint surfaces (Fig. **c**).

### Remarks

The same technique can be used when treating the segments of the lower thoracic area.

If the patient has painful arthrosis of the hip (coxarthrosis), one should not stabilize the patient by flexing his upper leg. Since good stabilization is important, however, the operator should place his forearm against the patient's pelvis as securely as the situation allows.

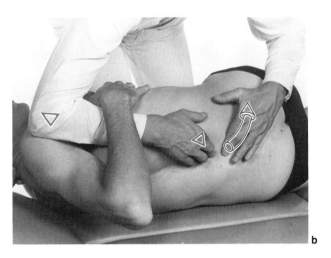

b

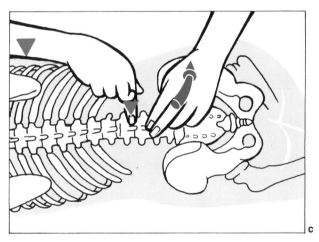

c

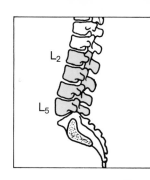

## Mobilization with Impulse (Thrust): Rotation and Side-Bending Restriction

### Indication (Fig. a)

*Zone of irritation:* L2, L3, L4, L5.
*Motion testing:* Segmental or regional motion restriction with hard endfeel.
*Pain:* Local or radiating to the gluteal region and legs.

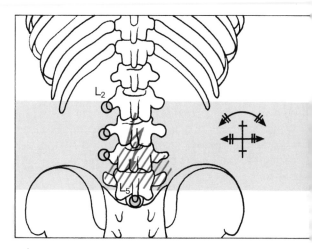

### Positioning

– The patient is in the side-lying position with his chest being approximately 10 cm away from the edge of the table.
– The pelvis is momentarily stabilized with the operator's hand that later will become the impulse hand. The patient's trunk is rotated so that his shoulder blades come to rest on the table.
– One of the patient's hands is placed under his head while the other hand rests on his chest.
– The operator presses on the patient's shoulder area, in particular in the pectoralis major muscle region, fixating the patient's trunk against the examination table (one should not press on the head of the humerus because it can be very painful).
– The patient's upper leg is passively flexed and the operator's knee is placed against the patient's poplitea (Fig. **b**). The operator's knee guides the patient's knee toward the floor until maximal rotation and localization in the lumbar spine are achieved (Fig. **b**).
– At this point, the operator allows the patient's shoulder to rotate until the operator makes floor contact with the stabilized leg. In this position the patient can be freely moved to and fro without great force.
– The middle finger supported by the index finger of the impulse hand is placed laterally over the spinous process of the restricted segment (Figs. **b, c**).

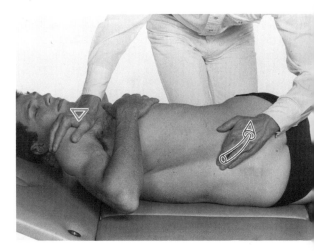

### Treatment Procedure

– Before the operator introduces a superiorly directed rotatory impulse force on the spinous process from a lateral approach, he introduces maximal rotation and side-bending by applying a steadily increasing force through his fixating hand (Fig. **c**).

## Mobilization without Impulse and NMT 2: Flexion Restriction

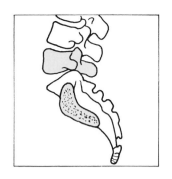

### Indications (Fig. a)

*Zone of irritation:* L5–S.

*Motion testing:* L5–S motion restriction.

*Remarks:* If there is hard endfeel during passive motion testing, one should apply mobilization without impulse. With soft endfeel during passive testing, one should apply NMT 2.

*Pain:* Chronic and localized.

*Muscle testing:* The erector spinae muscle is shortened in the lumbar region.

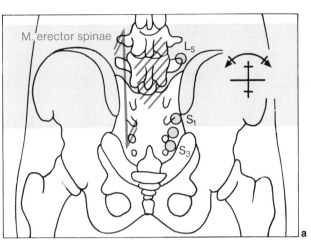

### Positioning

– Patient is in the side-lying position.
– The restricted segment is localized and engaged by rotating the thoracic and lumbar vertebrae above the restricted segment (slack is taken up to the restricted segment).
– With his arms, the operator fixates the thoracic and lumbar spine while his fingertips are placed over the spinous process of L5.
– His other hand is placed over the spinous process of S1 as well as the entire sacrum.
– The hip joint is flexed in order to prevent further motion in that joint. The patient's lower legs rest against the operator's body (Fig. **b**).

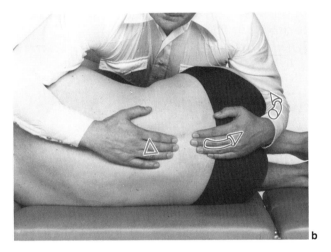

### Treatment Procedure

– Mobilization without impulse: The operator introduces traction to the spinous process of S1, thereby effecting passive mobilization and flexing the spinal segment. The hip joints are concurrently flexed as well (Fig. **b**).
– NMT 2: The restricted segment is brought to its pathologic barrier. Isometric extension is effected away from the motion barrier during inhalation (Fig. **c**).
– During the postisometric relaxation phase, the segment is then mobilized beyond the pathologic barrier while the patient exhales.

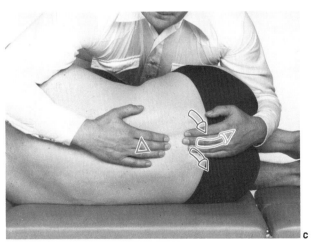

## Mobilization without Impulse and NMT 1: Anterior Motion Restriction

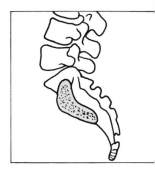

### Indication (Fig. a)

*Zone of irritation:* S1, S2, S3.

*Motion testing:* Sacroiliac joint (SIJ) motion restriction with hard endfeel.

*Pain:* Chronic and localized, sometimes radiating to the buttocks region and posterior thigh.

*Muscle testing:* The piriformis muscle is sometimes shortened, as are the hamstring muscles.

### Positioning

– Patient is prone.
– The operator places his hand over that half of the sacrum adjoining the restricted SIJ (Fig. **b**).

### Treatment Procedure

– Mobilization without impulse: anterior passive mobilization (Fig. **b**).
– NMT 1: With the sacrum stabilized, the patient lifts his pelvis off the table on the restricted side (the hip joint is slightly extended) (Fig. **c**).

### Remarks

One should avoid too great a lordotic curve in the lumbar spine when applying this active mobilization technique.

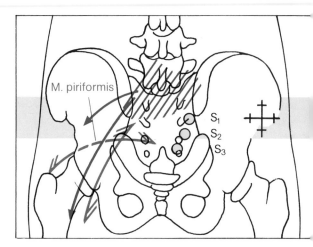

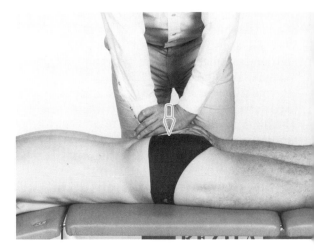

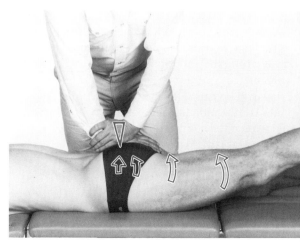

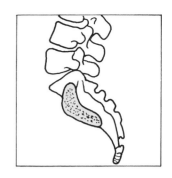

## Mobilization without Impulse and NMT 2: Anterior Motion Restriction

### Indication (Fig. a)

*Zone of irritation:* S1, S2, S3.

*Motion testing:* SIJ motion restriction.

*Pain:* Chronic and sometimes acute. Localized or radiating to the buttocks region and posterior thigh.

*Muscle testing:* The piriformis muscle may be shortened.

### Positioning

– Patient is supine.
– The hip joint on the restricted side is flexed and slightly adducted.
– The operator places his hand flat over the sacrum (Fig. **b**).

### Treatment Procedure

– Mobilization without impulse: The operator indirectly mobilizes the SIJ by applying a force on the patient's femur (the force is along the femur's axis) (Fig. **b**).
– NMT 2: optimal isometric contraction along the direction of the axis of the femur.
– During the postisometric phase, the joint is mobilized beyond the motion barrier (Fig. **c**).

### Remarks

This technique should only be used if there is no pain in the hip joint. If the piriformis muscle is shortened significantly, it should be stretched before mobilization is applied.

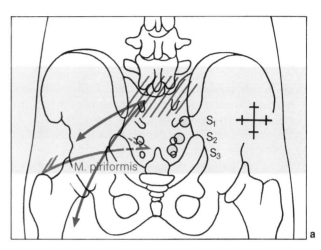

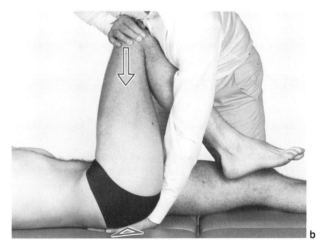

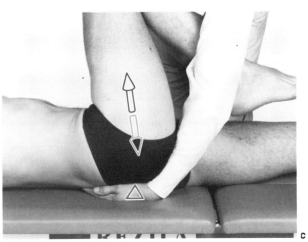

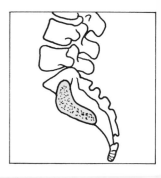

## Mobilization with Impulse (Thrust): Anterior and Inferior Motion Restriction

### Indication (Fig. a)

*Zone of irritation:* Sacrum, the entire region of the SIJ; exacerbated by provocative testing.

*Motion testing:* SIJ motion restriction with hard endfeel.

*Pain:* Low back pain occasionally radiating into the buttocks area, poplitea and heel.

### Positioning

- The patient is in the side-lying position close to the edge of the examination table with the restricted SIJ facing away from the table.
- The operator fixates the patient's pelvis with one hand. He grasps the patient's lower forearm, pulling the patient's shoulder toward him.
  He then rotates the upper shoulder away, introducing rotation to the thoracic spine, taking up the slack in the thoracic and lumbar spine.
- The patient is stabilized in this position via the operator fixating the shoulder or placing his elbows against the patient's axilla.
- The patient turns his eyes in the direction of rotation allowing reflexive relaxation of the back musculature.
- The restricted spinal segment can now be localized from inferior: the hand resting over the patient's pelvis introduces passive flexion to the hip through the upper thigh, bringing about flexion in the lumbar spine. The patient's foot of the upper leg is placed against the lower poplitea.
- The operator places his knee over the lateral aspect of the patient's flexed knee for further monitoring.
- With his forearm resting over the patient's greater trochanter, the operator's hand of the lower arm makes direct contact with the iliac crest that points away from the table (Fig. **b**).

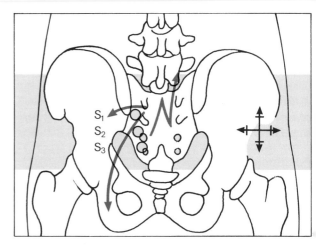

$S_1$
$S_2$
$S_3$

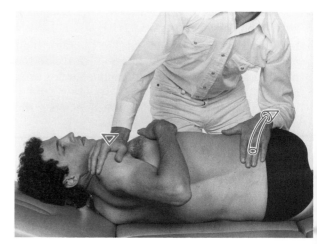

## Mobilization with Impulse (Thrust): Anterior and Inferior Motion Restriction (cont'd.)

### Treatment Procedure

– The impulse is effected through the iliac crest and the greater trochanter and is directed anteroinferiorly (Fig. **c**).

### Remarks

This mobilization technique has the advantage that the hand through which the impulse is effected does not touch the zone of irritation.

If the piriformis muscle is shortened, pain may already be apparent with positioning, in which case one should treat the piriformis muscle with NMT 2 mobilizing the SIJ.

If the patient has painful arthrosis of the hip (coxarthrosis), one should not stabilize the patient through the flexed upper leg (the leg that does not have table contact).

The operator places his forearm against the patient's pelvis as securely as the situation allows in order to guarantee the best stabilization possible.

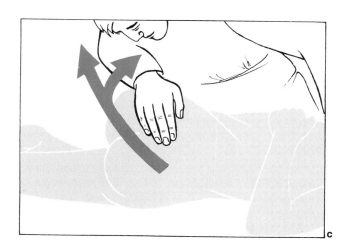

c

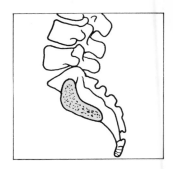

## Mobilization with Impulse: Anterior Motion Restriction

### Indication (Fig. a)

*Zone of irritation:* S2, the central portion of the SIJ, exacerbated by provocative testing.

*Motion testing:* SIJ motion restriction with hard end-feel.

*Pain:* Low back pain, occasionally radiating to the buttocks region, poplitea, and heel.

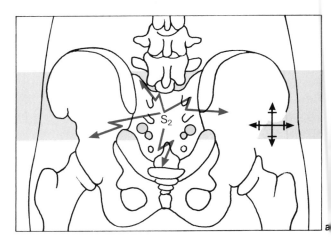

### Positioning

- The patient is in the side-lying position close to the edge of the examination table. The restricted SIJ faces the table.
- The operator fixates the patient's pelvis with one hand. He grasps the patient's lower forearm, pulling the patient's shoulder toward him.
- He then rotates the upper shoulder away, introducing rotation to the thoracic spine and slack is taken up in the thoracic and lumbar spine (barrier is found).
- The patient is stabilized in this position either via the operator fixating the shoulder or placing his elbows against the patient's axilla.
- The patient turns his eyes in the direction of rotation, allowing reflexive relaxation of the back musculature.
- The restricted spinal segment can now be localized and engaged from inferior: the hand resting over the patient's pelvis introduces passive flexion to the hip through the upper thigh, bringing about minimal but specific flexion in the lumbar spine. The patient's foot of the upper leg is placed against the lower poplitea.

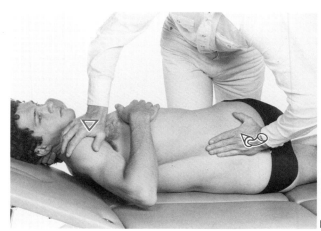

## Mobilization with Impulse: Anterior Motion Restriction (cont'd.)

– The operator places his knee over the lateral aspect of the patient's flexed poplitea for further monitoring.
– Lumbar spine and pelvis are rotated further in order to bring the anterior superior iliac spine in contact with the examination table.
– This may require that the previous thoracic spine rotation be somewhat reversed.
– The operator places the hypothenar of his lower hand on the half of the sacrum that points in the direction of the table (Figs. **b, c**).
– The pisiform bone rests over the zone of irritation.

### Treatment Procedure

– The impulse is directed anteriorly and should not contain a force component in the superior direction.

### Remarks

If pain occurs with positioning, one of the following causes may be responsible:
– The thoracic and lumbar spine are rotated too far.
– Fixation of the thoracic spine in rotation is too forceful.
– Significant shortening of the piriformis muscle, in which case the piriformis muscle should be treated with the NMT 2 technique before SIJ mobilization is undertaken.

If the patient has painful arthrosis of the hip (coxarthrosis) the patient should not be stabilized via the flexed upper leg. The operator places his forearm against the patient's pelvis as firmly as the situation allows in order to guarantee the best stabilization possible.

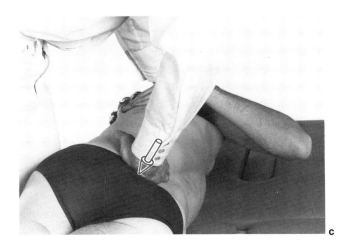

c

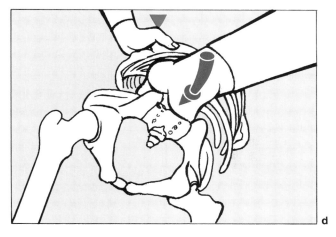

d

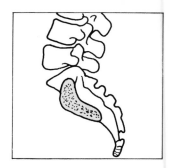

## Mobilization with Impulse (Superior-Axial): Flexion Motion Restriction

### Indication (Fig. a)

*Zone of irritation:* S1, in the upper portion of the SIJ, exacerbated by provocative testing.

*Motion testing:* SIJ motion restriction with hard end-feel.

*Pain:* Low back pain sometimes radiating to the buttocks, poplitea, and heel.

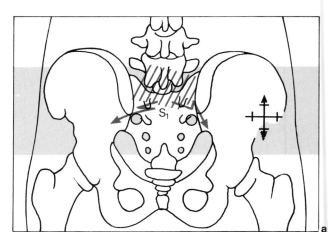

### Positioning

- The patient is in the side-lying position close to the edge of the examination table.
- The restricted SIJ faces the table.
- The operator fixates the patient's pelvis with one hand. He grasps the patient's forearm, pulling the shoulder toward him.
  He then rotates other shoulder away, introducing rotation to the thoracic spine and taking up the slack in the thoracic and lumbar spine.
- The patient is stabilized in this position either via the operator fixating the patient's shoulder or placing his elbows against the patient's axilla.
- The patient turns his eyes in the direction of rotation, allowing a reflexive relaxation of the back musculature.
- The restricted spinal segment can now be localized from inferior: the hand resting over the patient's pelvis now introduces passive flexion to the hip joint by bending the leg, subsequently bringing about flexion in the lumbar spine. The patient's foot of the upper leg rests against the lower poplitea.
- The operator places his knee over the lateral aspect of the patient's flexed knee for further monitoring.
- Lumbar spine and pelvis are further rotated so that the anterior superior iliac spine comes to rest on the table.
- It may be necessary to somewhat reverse the previously introduced thoracic-lumbar rotation.

## Mobilization with Impulse (Superior-Axial Traction): Flexion Motion Restriction (cont'd.)

– The operator then places the hypothenar of his inferior hand over the sacral half that points in the direction of the examination table (Figs. **b, c**).

### Treatment Procedure

– The impulse force is guided in a rather superior direction, which is often associated with an anterior force component as well (Fig. **c**).

### Remarks

If the patient reports pain with positioning, one or a combination of the following causes may be responsible:
– Insufficient or improper lumbar spine positioning. The lumbar spine may need to be flexed even further.
– Significant shortening of the piriformis muscle, in which case the piriformis muscle should be treated with the NMT 2 technique before SIJ mobilization is undertaken.

If the patient has painful arthrosis of the hip (coxarthrosis) the patient should not be stabilized by flexing the upper leg. The operator places his forearm against the patient's pelvis as firmly as the situation allows in order to guarantee the best stabilization possible.

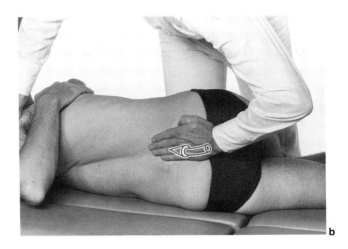

b

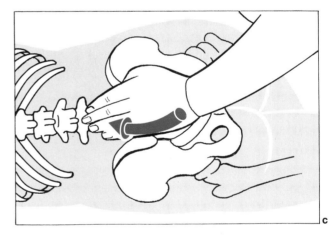

c

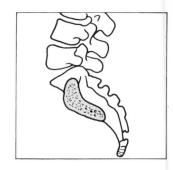

## Mobilization with Impulse (Thrust): Extension Restriction

### Indication (Fig. a)

*Zone of irritation:* S3, lower portion of the SIJ, provocative testing may exacerbate pain.

*Motion testing:* SIJ motion restriction with hard end-feel

*Pain:* Occasionally radiating to the buttocks, poplitea, and heel.

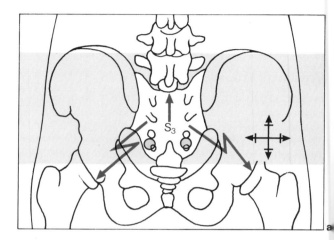

### Positioning

- The patient is in the side-lying position close to the edge of the examination table. The restricted SIJ faces the table.
- The operator fixates the patient's pelvis with one hand. He then grasps the patient's forearm, pulling the shoulder toward him.
- He then rotates the other shoulder away, introducing rotation to the thoracic spine and taking up the slack in the thoracic and lumbar spine.
- The patient is stabilized in this position either by the operator fixating the patient's shoulder or placing his elbows against the patient's axilla.
- The patient turns his eyes in the direction of rotation, allowing reflexive relaxation of the back musculature.
- The restricted spinal segment can now be localized and engaged from below: the hand resting over the patient's pelvis introduces passive flexion to the hip joint by bending the patient's leg, subsequently introducing flexion to the lumbar spine als well. The patient's foot of the upper leg is against the lower knee.
- The operator places his knee over the lateral aspect of the patient's bent knee for further monitoring.
- The operator places the hypothenar of his lower hand over the sacral half pointing toward the table, between the iliac crest and the medial sacral spine (Figs. **b, c**).

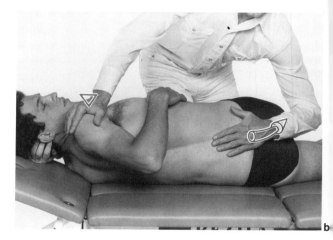

## Mobilization with Impulse (Thrust): Extension Restriction (cont'd.)

### Treatment Procedure

– The impulse is directed inferiorly and anteriorly. (Fig. **c**).

### Remarks

If the patient reports pain with positioning, one or a combination of the following causes may be responsible:
– The thoracic and lumbar spine have been rotated too far.
– Fixation of the thoracic spine in rotation is too forceful.
– Significant shortening of the piriformis muscle, in which case the muscle should be treated using the NMT 2 technique before SIJ mobilization.

If the patient has painful arthrosis of the hip (coxarthrosis) the patient should not be stabilized by flexing the upper leg. The operator places his forearm against the patient's pelvis as firmly as the situation allows, in order to guarantee the best stabilization possible.

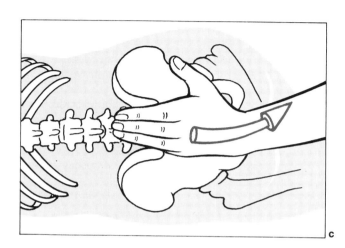

c

# SIJ

## NMT 1: Nutation Restriction

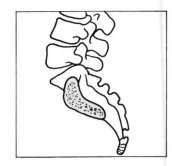

### Indication (Fig. a)

*Zones of irritation:* S1, S2, S3.

*Motion testing:* SIJ motion restriction with hard endfeel. The pubic bone on the same side as the restricted SIJ is more superior than the other side.

*Pain:* Chronic and localized; occasionally radiating into the buttocks region, medial and posterior thigh.

*Muscle testing:* The piriformis muscle is shortened, as may occasionally occur with the psoas major muscle.

### Positioning

- Patient is supine; lordotic curvature is reduced.
- The pelvis is stabilized on the nonrestricted side by introducing maximal flexion to the hip and knee joints.
- The operator fixates the leg on the restricted side by extending the thigh at the hip joint (Fig. **b**).

### Treatment Procedure

- The patient isometrically contracts the extended leg against equal resistance trying to perform flexion and adduction (Fig. **b**).

### Remarks

Muscle pull on the pubic bone mobilizes the sacroiliac joint indirectly.

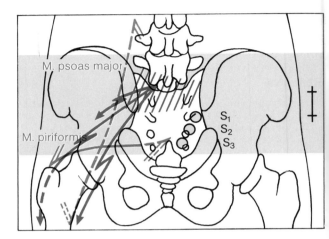

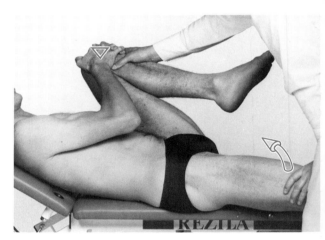

# SIJ

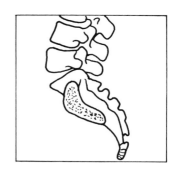

## NMT 1 and NMT 2: Nutation Restriction

### Indication (Fig. a)

*Zone of irritation:* S1, S2, S3.

*Motion testing:* SIJ motion restriction with hard endfeel.

*Pain:* Pain is either chronic or acute; localized and radiating into the buttocks region and posterior thigh.

*Muscle testing:* The piriformis muscle may be shortened.

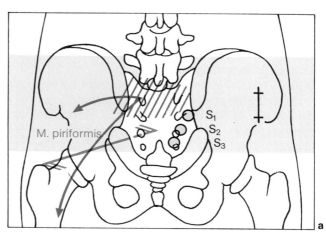

### Positioning

- Patient is in the side-lying position.
- The restricted sacroiliac joint points away from the table.
- The pelvis is stablized by introducing passive flexion to the leg on the restricted side.
- The operator fixates the sacrum with his lateral hand margin.

*Remarks:* The lumbar spine should be slightly flexed, but movement in the lumbar spine should be avoided (Fig. **b**).

### Treatment Procedure

- NMT 1: Active extension of the pelvis against the resisting force applied at the sacrum (Fig. **b**).
- NMT 2: Maximal isometric contraction in the direction of extension (synchronous with inhalation).
- During the postisometric relaxation phase, the sacrum is passively mobilized in an anteroinferior direction (synchronous with exhalation) (Fig. **c**).

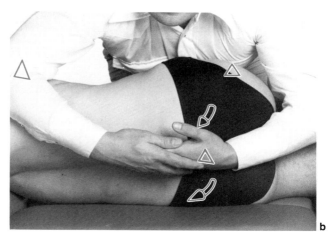

### Remarks

If the patient reacts to this mobilization procedure with pain in the lumbar spine one or a combination of the following causes may be responsible:

- Unsatisfactory lumbar spine positioning
- Insufficient sacrum fixation
- Severely shortened piriformis muscle, in which case the muscle should be stretched before this mobilization procedure.

Isometric pelvic extension requires that the patient develop a sense of how to perform this movement properly. It is often necessary to teach the patient proper technique by using passive and guided, resistive movements.

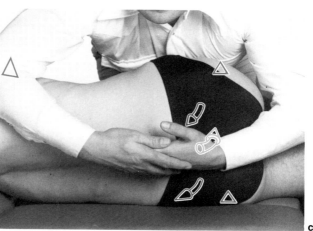

# Rib I

## Mobilization without Impulse: Exhalation (Inferior) Restriction

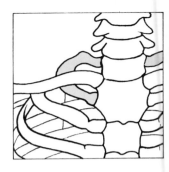

### Indication (Fig. a)

*Zone of irritation:* Rib I.

*Motion testing:* Rib I motion restriction during exhalation with hard endfeel.

*Pain:* Chronic in the shoulder region. Paresthesias affecting the arm during sleep at night.

*Muscle testing:* Shortening of the scalene muscles and occasionally the descending portion of the trapezius muscle.

### Positioning

– Patient is seated.
– The operator stabilizes with his thigh and elbow the shoulder on the side opposite to that of the incriminated rib.
– He fixates the patient's head and stabilizes the cervical spine in the side-bent position toward the side of mobilization (Fig. **b**).
– The fingers are placed over the first rib, with the thumb at the neck.

### Treatment Procedure

– Passive mobilization in an inferior and medial direction during exhalation (Fig. **b**).

### Remarks

If the hand exerts too great a pressure over the brachial plexus, paresthesias in the arm may become apparent.

One should not press against the transverse processes of C7 and T1.

One should not increase the cervical spine side-bending during the mobilization procedure.

If there is concurrent hypomobility and a zone of irritation in the cervicothoracic junction, one should treat it before treating the first rib, since finger placement for treatment of the first rib can bring the fingers into contact with the zone of irritation in the cervicothoracic junction.

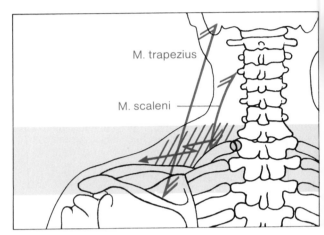

M. trapezius

M. scaleni

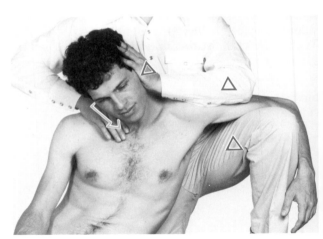

# Rib I

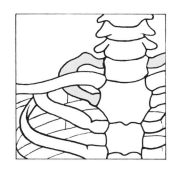

## Mobilization without Impulse: Exhalation (Inferior) Restriction

### Indication: (Fig. a)

*Zone of irritation:* Rib I.

*Motion testing:* Rib I motion restriction during exhalation with hard endfeel.

*Pain:* Chronic in the shoulder region. Occasional paresthesias in the arm during sleep at night.

*Muscle testing:* Shortening of the scalene muscles and the descending portion of the trapezius muscle.

### Positioning

- Patient is supine.
- Legs are flexed.
- Passive cervical spine side-bending is toward the side of mobilization.
- The fingers and thumb, forming a vicelike grip, follow the course of the first rib (Fig. **b**).

### Treatment Procedure

- Passive mobilization in the inferior and medial direction during exhalation (Fig. **b**).

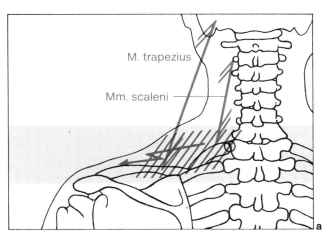

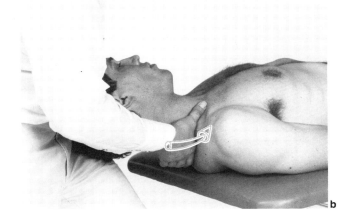

# Ribs VI to XII

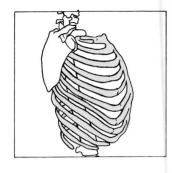

## Mobilization without Impulse: Anterior Rib Motion Restriction

### Indication (Fig. a)

*Zone of irritation:* Ribs VI, VII, VIII, IX, X, XI, XII.

*Motion testing:* Rib motion restriction. Possible restriction of regional thorax mobility.

*Pain:* Acute or chronic and often associated with respiratory movement. Pain may be localized or runs along the rib toward the sternum.

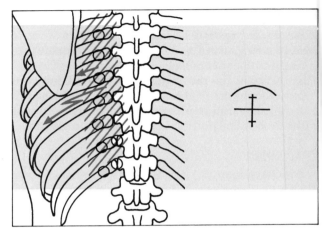

### Positioning

- Patient is prone.
- The operator fixates the incriminated rib at the costal angle with his pisiform bone.
- The other hand is placed over the anterior iliac spine (Fig. **b**).

### Treatment Procedure

- The involved rib is passively mobilized by the operator rotating the patient's pelvis and lumbar spine to the level of the involved rib.

### Remarks

This technique may be difficult to apply when there are additional painful dysfunctions in the:
- Lumbar spine
- Sacroiliac joints
- Lower thoracic spine

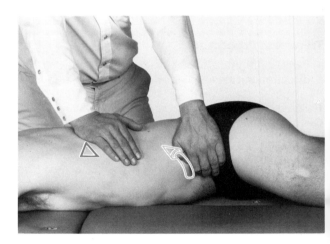

# Rib I

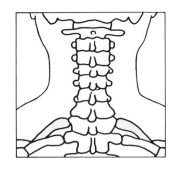

## Mobilization with Impulse (Thrust): Inferior-Anterior Rib Motion Restriction

### Indication (Fig. a)

*Zone of irritation:* Rib I.
*Motion testing:* First rib motion restriction with hard endfeel during exhalation.
*Pain:* Localized or possibly radiating toward the arms associated with paresthesias (during the night).

### Positioning

– Patient is seated.
– The shoulder on the noninvolved side is stabilized by the operator's thigh and elbow.
– The patient's head is side-bent to the involved side and then fixated.
– The metacarpal head of the second finger of the other hand makes contact with the first rib (Fig. **b**).

### Treatment Procedure

– During exhalation, an impulse is directed inferiorly and medially (Fig. **c**).

### Remarks

Caveat:
– The hand through which the impulse is effected may cause paresthesias when too great a pressure is exerted on the brachial plexus.

Quite frequently there is vertebral restriction associated with rib restriction. If this is the case, one should mobilize the thoracic spinal segment before mobilizing the rib.

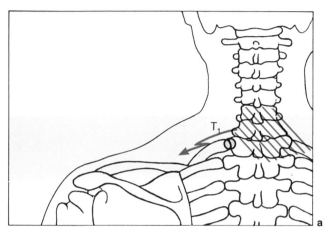

a

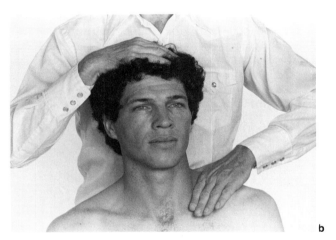

b

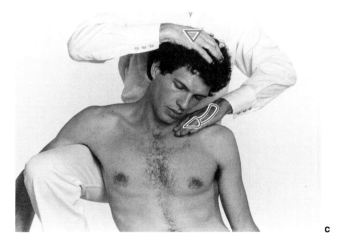

c

# Ribs II to VI

## Mobilization with Impulse (Thrust): Anterior Motion Restriction

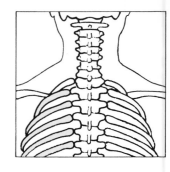

### Indication (Fig. a)

*Zone of irritation:* Rib II, III, IV, V, VI.

*Motion testing:* Rib motion restriction with hard end-feel.

Diminished "bucket handle" type of breathing on the involved side.

*Pain:* Related to the respiratory movement. Pain is along the course of the rib toward the sternum; pain may be localized. Occasional shoulder or arm pain.

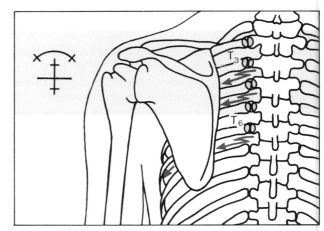

### Positioning

- The patient is supine with the arms crossed in front of his chest.
- The operator stands opposite to the side that is to be mobilized. He rotates the patient toward him, placing the thenar eminence over the costal angle of the restricted rib (Fig. **b**).
- The patient is then rotated back to the supine position.

### Treatment Procedure

- During exhalation, the operator effects an anterior impulse force on the restricted rib through the patient's crossed arms.

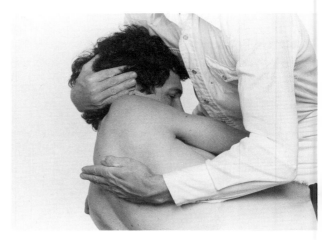

### Remarks

Quite frequently there is associated hypomobility in a thoracic spinal segment when the respective rib is restricted. In this case, one should mobilize the thoracic spinal segment before mobilizing the rib itself.

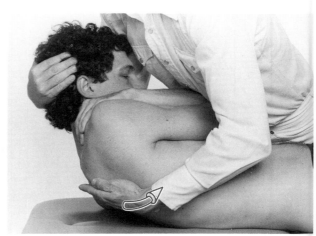

# Ribs VI to XII

## Mobilization with Impulse (Thrust): Anterior and Lateral Motion Restriction

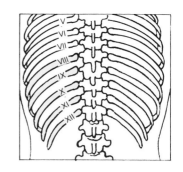

### Indication (Fig. a)

*Zone of irritation:* Ribs VI, VII, VIII, IX, X, XI, XII.

*Motion testing:* Rib motion restriction with hard end-feel.

Diminished "bucket handle" type of respiration on the involved side.

*Pain:* Related to respiratory movement. The distribution is along the course of the rib radiating to the sternum. Pain may be localized.

### Positioning

– Patient is prone with the thoracic spine slightly flexed.
– The operator standing at the patient's side fixates with his hypothenar the involved rib in the region of the costal angle.
– The other hand is placed over the anterior iliac spine on the side of the involved rib.
– The anterior iliac spine is lifted off the table, introducing rotation to the lumbar spine in order to bring it to its respective barrier (Fig.**b**).

### Treatment Procedure

– During exhalation, the impulse force is effected through the hypothenar in the anteroinferior direction (Fig. **b**).

### Remarks

– If there is associated pain in the lumbar spine or the sacroiliac region, one should refrain from using this technique.

Quite frequently, there is hypomobility in the thoracic spinal segment when the respective rib is restricted. In this case, one should mobilize the thoracic spinal segments before mobilizing the rib.

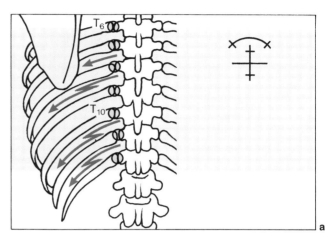

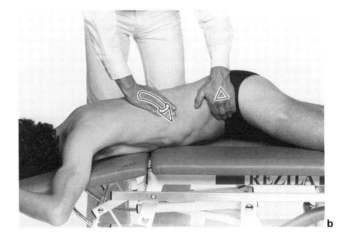

# Ribs V to XII

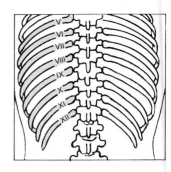

## Mobilization with Impulse (Thrust): Anterior-Inferior Motion Restriction

### Indication (Fig. a)

*Zone of irritation:* Ribs V, VI, VII, VIII, IX, X, XI, XII.

*Motion testing:* Rib motion restriction with hard end-feel.

Diminished "bucket handle" type of respiration on the involved side.

*Pain:* Related to respiratory movement. Pain distribution is along the course of the involved rib radiating to the sternum. Pain may be localized. Occasional shoulder-arm pain.

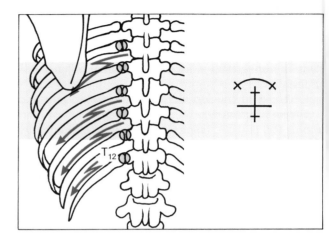

### Positioning

– Patient is supine with the arms internally rotated and the cervical spine slightly flexed.
– The operator places his thenar eminence broadly over the costal angle of the involved rib.
– He places the other hand flat over the patient's thorax opposite to the side of the involved rib for monitoring purposes (Fig. **b**).

### Treatment Procedure

– During exhalation, an anteroinferior impulse force is effected to the rib (Fig. **b**).

### Remarks

Quite frequently one may find restriction in the associated thoracic spinal segment when the rib is restricted. If this is the case, one should mobilize the thoracic spinal segment before mobilizing the rib.

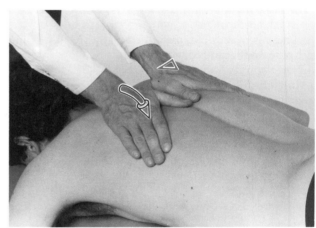

# Ribs II to XII

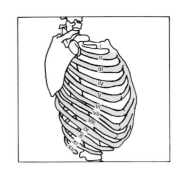

## Mobilization without Impulse and NMT 1: Anterior Rib Motion Restriction

### Indications (Fig. a)

*Zone of irritation:* Ribs II to XII.

*Motion testing:* Rib motion restriction with possible restriction of regional thorax mobility.

*Pain:* Acute or chronic; often dependent on respiratory movement. Pain may be localized or course along the rib toward the sternum.

### Positioning

– The patient is prone with the arms maximally internally rotated at the shoulder. The thoracic spine is slightly flexed.
– The operator places his hand over the costal angle of the involved rib (Fig. **b**).

### Treatment Procedure

– Mobilization without impulse: Passive rib mobilization in the anterior direction (Fig. **b**).
– NMT 1: As the patient deeply inhales, the rib is fixated and held at the costal angle, introducing mobilization (Fig. **c**).

### Remarks

To avoid rib fractures, especially in older patients, one should carefully dose the stabilizing force.

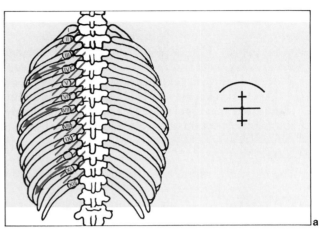

a

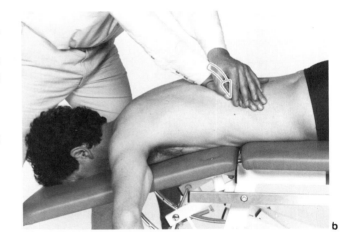

b

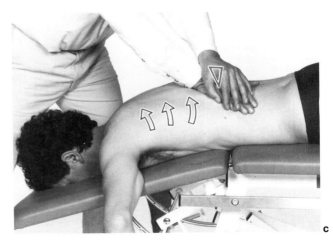

c

# Ribs IV to XII

## Mobilization without Impulse and NMT 1: Anterior Motion Restriction

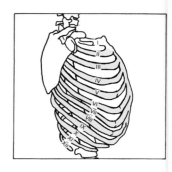

### Indications (Fig. a)

*Zone of irritation:* Ribs IV through XII.

*Motion testing:* Rib motion restriction with rather hard endfeel.

Thorax mobility may be restricted regionally.

*Pain:* Acute or chronic and frequently dependent on respiratory movement. Pain courses along the rib toward the sternum or may be localized.

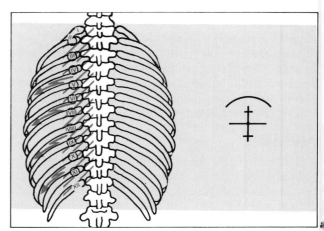

### Positioning

– The patient is supine with his legs flexed and arms crossed over his chest.
– The operator standing on the noninvolved side passively rotates the patient toward him, placing his thenar eminence over the costal angle of the restricted rib (Fig. **b**).

### Treatment Procedure

– Mobilization without impulse: the operator mobilizes the rib by passively rotating the patient away from him, with the thenar eminence providing the resistant force (Fig. **c**).
– NMT 1: the involved rib is held stationary at its movement endpoint (barrier) by the operator's thenar eminence and is mobilized while the patient deeply inhales (Fig. **d**).

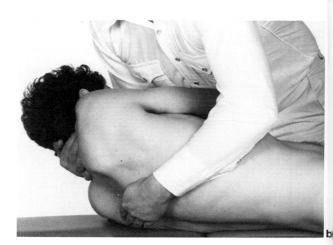

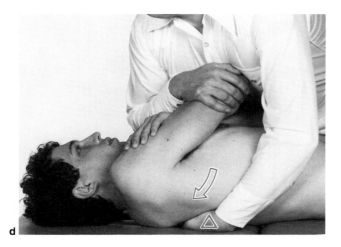

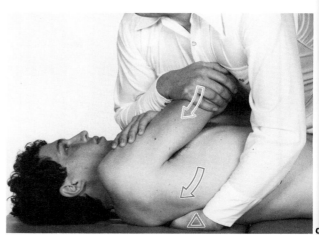

# Ribs IV to XII

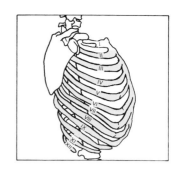

## NMT 2: Anterior Motion Restriction

### Indication (Fig. a)

*Zone of irritation:* Ribs IV to XII.

*Motion testing:* Rib motion restriction with rather hard endfeel.

*Pain:* Acute or chronic and related to the respriatory movement. Along the rib to the sternum or local pain.

### Positioning

- The patient is in the side-lying position.
- The thoracic spine is rotated from superior down to the level of the incriminated rib. The operator places either his index or middle finger over the restricted rib, with the rest of the hand resting broadly over the patient's thorax (Fig. **b**).

### Treatment Procedure

- The involved rib is brought to its barrier and held there.
- The patient first inhales deeply, and then while he exhales the rib is passively mobilized in an anteroinferior direction (Fig. **b**).

Patient's gaze:
- During inhalation: towards the restricted side.
- During exhalation: away from the restricted side.

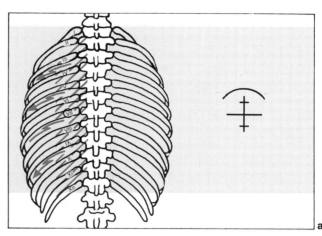

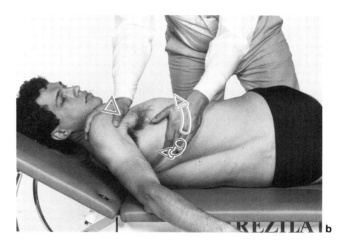

# Sternocleidomastoid Muscle

## NMT 2

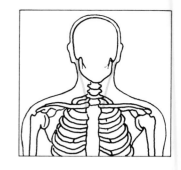

### Indication (Fig. a)

*Motion testing:* Cervical spine side-bending and rotation restriction; soft endfeel.
  Thorax mobility i.e. "pumphandle" movement in upper ribs is often restricted, especially in patients with obstructive lung disease or emphysema.
*Pain:* There is occasional pain in the cervical spine and arm (cervicobrachialgia), which is often seen in association with segmental dysfunctions in the cervical or thoracic spines.
*Muscle testing:* The sternocleidomastoid muscle is shortened. Frequently, the descending portion of the trapezius muscle and the scalene muscles are shortened as well.

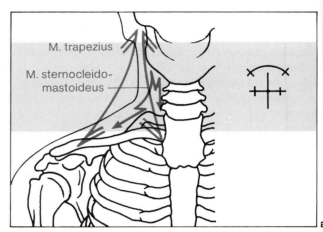

M. trapezius
M. sternocleido-mastoideus

### Positioning

– Patient is supine with his head beyond the examination table and resting on the operator's thighs (operator is seated).
– The muscle is maximally stretched by introducing passive cervical spine rotation and side-bending to the opposite side (Fig. **b**).

### Treatment Procedure

– The shortened sternocleidomastoid muscle is contracted isometrically during inhalation, with the patient looking in a superior direction.
– During the postisometric relaxation phase, the muscle is passively stretched, primarily by accentuating the side-bending component, less the rotation component. This occurs during exhalation with the patient looking inferiorly (Fig. **b**).

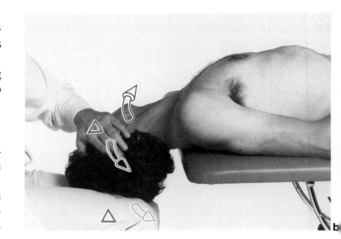

### Remarks

The individual stretching steps are rather small.
The treatment procedure should be immediately terminated when signs of a possible vertebral artery compression develop, as expressed by vertigo, nausea, or spontaneous nystagmus.
This stretching technique should only be applied after any segmental dysfunction has been improved with the appropriate techniques so that there is no longer any hard endfeel present.

# Scalene Muscles

## NMT 2

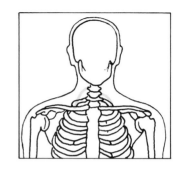

### Indication (Fig. a)

*Motion testing:* Restricted mobility of the first rib and the upper thorax during exhalation. Restricted cervical spine extension and side-bending with soft endfeel.

*Pain:* Chronic cervicobrachialgia with frequent paresthesias during the night. Occasionally, may the classic signs of the scalenus anticus syndrome (both neurologic and vascular) are found.

*Muscle testing:* The scalene muscles are shortened and often the descending portion of the trapezius muscle as well as the sternocleidomastoid muscle are shortened.

*Note:* In many cases there is prominent upper thorax (sternal) respiration especially in combination with obstructive lung disease or emphysema.

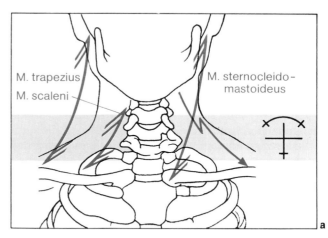

### Positioning

– Patient is supine with his head beyond the examination table and resting on the operator's thigh (operator seated).
– Maximal stretch is introduced by extending and side-bending the cervical spine and rotating the neck to the opposite side (Fig. **b**).

### Treatment Procedure

– The shortened scalene muscles are isometrically contracted as much as possible (during inhalation, upward gaze).
– During the postisometric relaxation phase and with the cervical spine fixated, the first rib and the clavicle are pushed inferiorly (during exhalation and downward gaze).
– This brings about further extension and side-bending to the cervical spine (Fig. **b**).

*Note:* While the operator stretches the muscle, he should also introduce slight traction to the cervical spine.

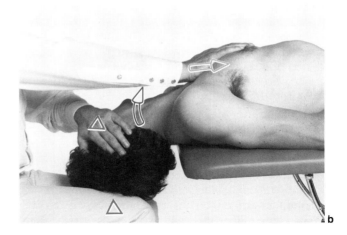

### Remarks

The treatment procedure should be terminated if with positioning or during the mobilization procedure there appear signs of possible vertebral artery compression or sympathicus nerve irritation, i.e., dizziness, nausea, or nystagmus. If there is concurrent first rib restriction or segmental dysfunction in the cervicothoracic spine, these areas should be treated first in order to guarantee proper stretch in the absence of reflexive endfeel.
If the descending portion of the trapezius muscle is also shortened it should be stretched before the scalene muscles.

# Trapezius Muscle, Descending Portion

## NMT 2

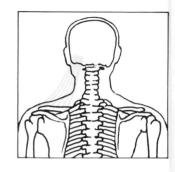

### Indication (Fig. a)

*Motion testing:* Decreased cervical spine side-bending with soft endfeel.

*Pain:* Chronic pain occurs in the neck region, which may radiate toward the occiput and arms.

*Muscle testing:* The descending portion of the trapezius muscle is shortened, with characteristic pain when stretched.

Often the medial shoulder blade fixator muscles are weak.

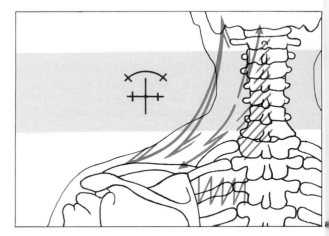

### Positioning

- The patient is supine with his head beyond the examination table.
- The operator places one hand over the occiput while the other hand is placed over the patient's shoulder.
- Passive maximal side-bending with rotation of the cervical spine is introduced (usually in the direction opposite to the side of involvement (Fig. **b**).

### Treatment Procedure

- The operator provides the resistant force to the patient's shoulder.
- Optimal isometric contraction of the trapezius muscle, descending portion.
- During the postisometric relaxation phase the muscle is passively stretched by mobilizing the shoulder girdle inferiorly and laterally (Fig. **b**).
- The cervical spine is carried to its new barrier, and treatment can be repeated, realizing the stretch of the muscle.

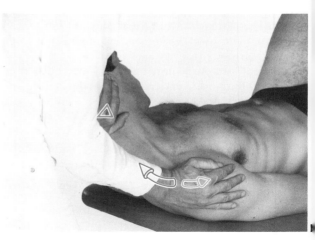

*Note:* One should utilize some traction to the cervical spine when applying this maneuver. This technique can also be carried out with the patient in the sitting position (Fig. **c**).

### Remarks

If there is dizziness or pain with positioning or during the treatment procedure itself, the cervical spine and the first rib should be examined for segmental dysfunctions and, if necessary, those areas should be treated before applying this technique.

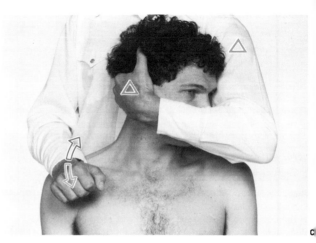

# Levator Scapulae Muscle

## NMT 2

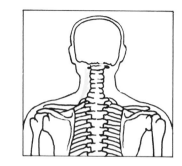

### Indication (Fig. a)

*Motion testing:* Diminished upper cervical spine flexion with soft endfeel. Increased chin-to-sternum distance, often in association with rotation and inclination restriction in the C1–C2 or C2–C3 segments.

*Pain:* Chronic pain in the neck region.
   Often the pain radiates toward the occiput and the region between the scapulae.

*Muscle testing:* The levator scapulae muscle is shortened with characteristic pain on stretching.
   There is often associated suboccipital muscle shortening.

*Palpation:* It is often difficult to test muscle length.
   A shortened levator scapulae muscle exhibits both muscle tension (texture) changes and crepitations that can be ascertained by palpating the distal muscle portion.

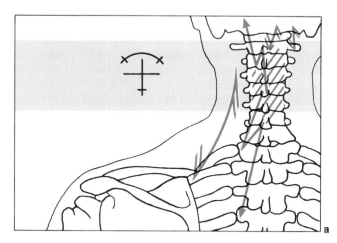

### Positioning

– The patient is supine with the head beyond the examination table.
– The operator places one hand flat over the patient's occiput. The other hand is placed over the patient's elbow after having introduced maximal abduction and external rotation to the arm, locking the shoulder joint in this position.
– The cervical spine is flexed (inclined) and rotated to the opposite side, introducing maximal stretch to the muscle.

### Treatment Procedure

– The operator provides the resistant force to the patient's elbow.
– Optimal isometric contraction of the levator scapulae muscle is performed by the patient.
– During the postisometric relaxation phase, passive stretch is introduced by pushing the scapula inferiorly and laterally via the patient's arm.
– Starting from this new barrier, the stretching technique is repeated.

*Note:* Some traction should be applied to the cervical spine during the entire procedure.

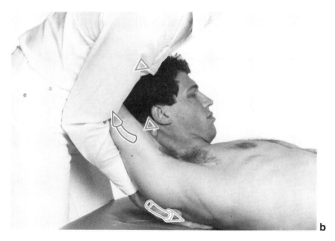

### Remarks

If dizziness or pain appear with positioning or during the treatment procedure itself, one should terminate this maneuver and examine and treat the cervical spine if indicated: In the case of segmental dysfunction in the upper cervical spine such a dysfunction should be treated before the levator scapulae muscle is stretched.

# Pectoralis Major Muscle

## NMT 2

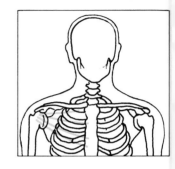

### Indication (Fig. a)

*Motion testing:* Diminished arm abduction and external rotation with soft endfeel.

*Pain:* Pain occurs in the axilla at the end of arm abduction and external rotation. The insertions at the ribs are quite tender to palpation.

*Muscle testing:* The pectoralis major muscle is shortened with characteristic pain on stretch. Often, there is simultaneous shortening of the descending portion of the trapezius muscle and weakening of the medial shoulder blade fixator muscles.

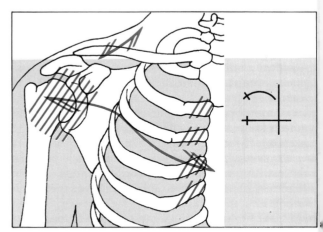

### Positioning

– The patient is supine, lying close to the edge of the examination table.
– The operator stands at the patient's head fixating the patient's thorax with one hand and the forearm.
– The other hand is placed over the patient's arm, introducing abduction and external rotation in order to stretch the muscle maximally (Fig. **b**).

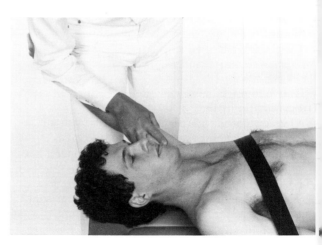

### Treatment Procedure

– The operator provides the resistant force to the patient's arm.
– Optimal isometric contraction of the pectoralis major muscle is performed by the patient.
– During the postisometric relaxation phase, the arm is passively abducted, utilizing additional slight traction. The increase in mobility is correlated to the extent of the stretch of the muscle (Fig. **b**).

### Remarks

If there is painful joint disease affecting the humeroscapular joint, this technique should not be utilized until later in the course of treatment.

Modification: The operator places one hand broadly over the muscle belly, which during the postisometric relaxation phase is moved along its longitudinal axis (Fig. **c**). Even though this technique contradicts the treatment principles delineated for NMT 2, it is, in addition to possibly using NMT 3, the only technique that allows pectoralis major muscle stretching in the presence of a painful shoulder joint (Fig. **c**).

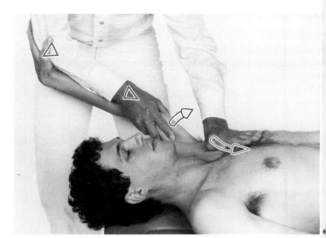

# Erector Spinae Muscle in the Lumbar Area

## NMT 2

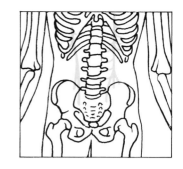

### Indication (Fig. a)

*Motion testing:* Lumbar spine flexion and side-bending restriction with soft endfeel.

*Pain:* Pain is localized to the patient's back; can be chronic or acute and may radiate into the legs.

*Muscle testing:* The erector spinae muscle is shortened and its contours become rather prominent. The psoas major and quadratus lumborum muscles are often shortened and the abdominal muscles are weak. Furthermore, there may coexist a segmental dysfunction in the lumbar spine or the pelvis, and there may be concurrent hip joint disease.

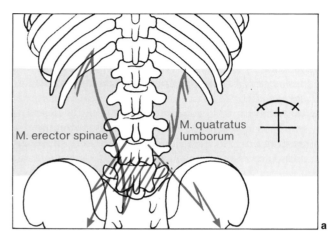

M. erector spinae    M. quatratus lumborum

### Positioning

– The patient is in the side-lying position.
– The muscle is maximally stretched by flexing the lumbar spine, hip, and knee joints.
– The operator places his hands flat over the sacrum and spinous processes in the midlumbar spine (Fig.**c**).

### Treatment Procedure

– During inhalation the erector spinae muscle is isometrically contracted to optimum.
– During the postisometric relaxation phase, passive stretch is introduced by further flexing the lumbar spine (traction at the sacrum).
– Since the hip joints are also increasingly flexed, pelvic flexion is also introduced, in turn, providing further stretch indirectly (Fig. **b**).

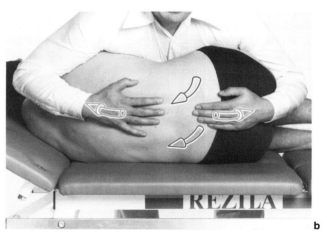

### Remarks

The patient may simply contract the erector spinae muscles, and so it is necessary to teach not know how to and practice the isometric contraction process before the operator advances to use the technique described here. Simple hip extension or pelvis extension are not sufficient.

# Quadratus Lumborum Muscle

**NMT 2**

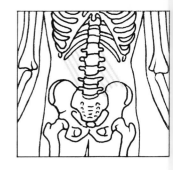

### Indication (Fig. a)

*Motion testing:* Restricted lumbar spine side-bending with soft endfeel.

*Pain:* Flank pain, which is often chronic.

*Muscle testing:* The quadratus lumborum muscle is shortened.

In addition, the erector spinae muscle in the lumbar area is shortened, and there may be segmental dysfunctions in the lumbar spine, and pelvis or associated disorders of the hip.

### Positioning

– The patient lies on his nonaffected side. The muscle is maximally stretched by passively side-bending the patient (patient is placed over a soft roll).
– The pelvis is stabilized by flexing the leg that is in contact with the table.
– The operator places his hands flat over the pelvic crest and the thorax in the area of ribs VI–X along the axillary line (Fig. **b**).

### Treatment Procedure

– During deep inhalation, the shortened quadratus lumborum muscle is isometrically contracted to optimum.
– During the postisometric relaxation phase, the muscle is passively stretched by pushing the pelvic crest and the thorax in opposite direction during inhalation (Fig. **b**).

*Note:* With each stretching process, there is a stepwise increase in side-bending movement, and the procedure is repeated from the newly engaged barrier.

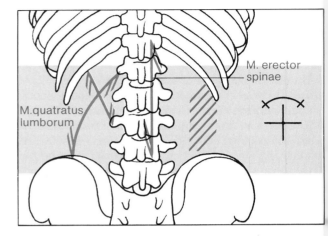

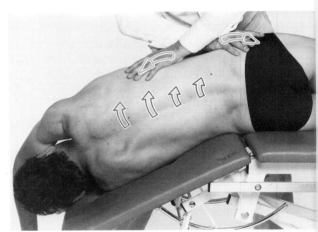

# Tensor Fasciae Latae Muscle

## NMT 2

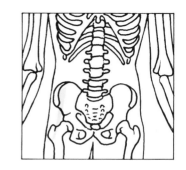

### Indication (Fig. a)

*Motion testing:* Diminished adduction of the leg with soft endfeel.
  (The skin on the lateral portion of the thigh retracts as well.)
*Pain:* Pain at the lateral side of the thigh. Pain can be elicited by palpating the insertion of the muscle.
*Muscle testing:* The tensor fasciae latae muscle is shortened with characteristic pain when stretched.

### Positioning

- The patient lies on the involved side.
- The pelvis is stabilized by having the patient flex hip and knee on the nontreatment side.
  It is recommended that a belt be utilized for further fixation of the pelvis.
- The operator grasps the extended leg (the leg facing the examination table), with one hand placed at the distal end of the thigh and the other at the distal end of the lower leg.
- Passive adduction is introduced, up to the point where the muscle is stretched maximally (Fig. **b**).

### Treatment Procedure

- The operator provides a resistant force with both hands.
- The tensor faciae latae muscle is isometrically contracted to optimum.
- During the postisometric relaxation phase, the operator follows the path of greatest adduction possible.
- Starting from this new position, the technique is repeated, and the mobility gain is correlated with the extent of muscle stretch effected.

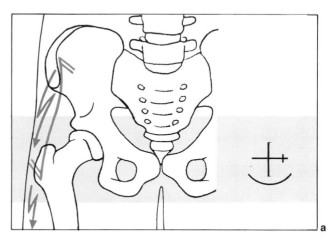

a

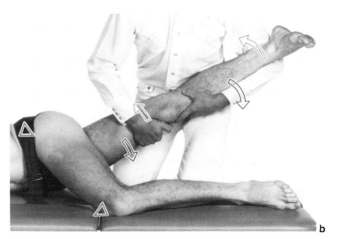

b

# Iliopsoas Muscle

### NMT 2

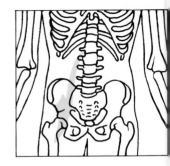

### Indication (Fig. a)

*Motion testing:* Diminished hip extension with soft endfeel, with the lumbar lordosis flattened (diminished lordosis).

*Pain:* Pain is rather diffuse in the lower abdominal and inguinal region.

*Muscle testing:* The iliopsoas muscle is shortened with characteristic pain when stretched. The erector spinae muscle in the lumbar area is often shortened, and the abdominal muscles are often weak.

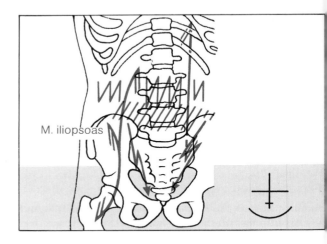

M. iliopsoas

### Positioning

- The patient is standing at the end of the examination table, which should be level with the patient's ischium.
- The nontreatment leg is maximally flexed and held up by the patient.
- The thoracic and lumbar spines are both flexed (Fig. **b**).
- The operator then places his hands on the patient's thoracic area and flexed leg and subsequently guides the patient passively into the supine position. The upper thoracic and cervical spine are supported by a roll while the lumbar lordosis remains flattened.
- The operator fixates the patient's flexed leg with his body and places one hand broadly over the distal area of the patient's thigh.
- Passive hip extension to the barrier is introduced (Fig.**c**).

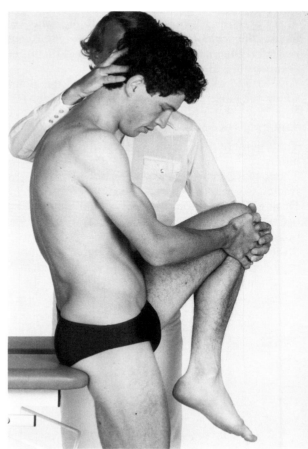

# Iliopsoas Muscle (cont'd.)

## NMT 2

### Treatment Procedure

- The operator provides the resistant force at the patient's thigh.
- The iliopsoas muscle is then isometrically contracted to optimum. During the postisometric relaxation phase, passive stretch is introduced by increasing hip extension (Fig. **c**). Starting from this new position, the technique is repeated, and the mobility gain can be correlated with the amount of stretch in the muscle.

### Remarks

If pain appears in the lumbar spine with this procedure, it might be the result of malpositioning, or one should employ the stretching with the patient prone (Fig. **d**).

### Positioning

- Patient is prone.
- The pelvis is fixated with the operator's hand and a belt.
- Passive hip extension to the barrier is introduced.

### Treatment Procedure

- The operator provides the resistant force at the patient's thigh.
- Optimal isometric contraction of the iliopsoas muscle is introduced. During the postisometric relaxation phase, passive stretch is introduced by increasing hip extension (Fig. **d**).

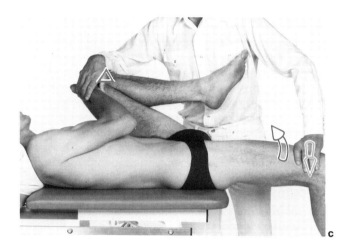

c

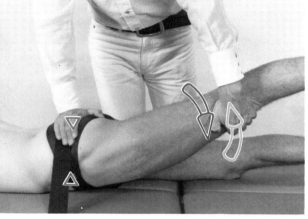

d

# Piriformis Muscle

## NMT 2

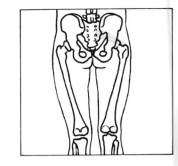

### Indication (Fig. a)

*Motion testing:* With the hip flexed, thigh adduction and external rotation are diminished; soft endfeel.

*Pain:* Chronic; localized or sometimes radiating to the posterior thigh. There is pain at the end of adduction and internal rotation of the leg. Pain occurs in the piriformis muscle on palpation.

*Muscle testing:* The piriformis muscle is shortened with characteristic pain when stretched.

### Positioning

- The patient is supine and the pelvis is stabilized either with a belt or by the operator.
- With the hip flexed approximately 70°, the thigh is adducted maximally, in order to evaluate the degree of piriformis muscle stretch possible (Fig. c).

### Treatment Procedure

- The operator's body provides the resistant force at the patient's thigh.
- The piriformis muscle is isometrically contracted to optimum.
- During the postisometric relaxation phase, the leg is passively adducted (Fig. c). Starting from this new position, the procedure is repeated, and the mobility gain can be correlated with the extent of muscle stretch effected.

### Remarks

If pain appears in the inguinal region while stretching the muscle, hip flexion should be reduced.

If pain appears in the sacroiliac joint region, there may be sacroiliac joint dysfunction, which should be treated before this procedure is applied. It is often difficult to differentiate between a tender piriformis muscle and pain secondary to the sciatic nerve.

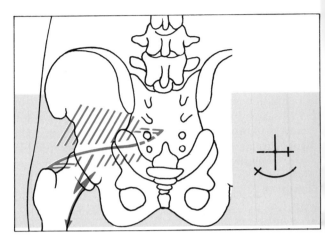

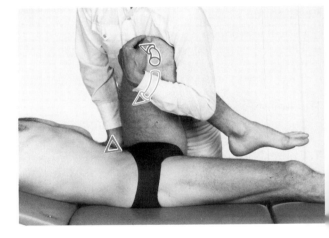

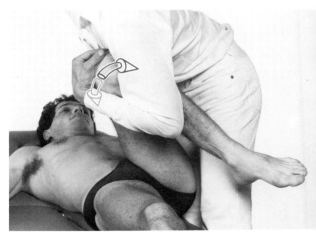

# Rectus Femoris Muscle

## NMT 2

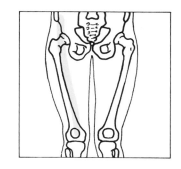

### Indication (Fig. a)

*Motion testing:* With the patient prone and the hip joint extended maximally, knee flexion is diminished with abrupt elastic endfeel. Pelvis flexion may increase with increasing passive knee flexion.

*Pain:* Localized to the anterior portion of the thigh, sometimes radiating to the patella.

*Muscle testing:* The rectus femoris muscle is shortened with typical pain when stretched.

Often the vastus medialis muscle is weak, and the erector spinae muscle in the lumbar area is shortened.

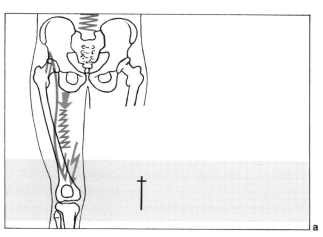

a

### Positioning

- The patient is prone and the pelvis is fixated with a belt.
- Utilizing passive knee flexion, one determines how much this muscle can be stretched.
- One of the operator's hands monitors pelvic movement. The other hand is placed on the anterior portion of the thigh, and the arm is placed against the patient's foreleg, stabilizing flexion and rotation (Fig. **b**).

### Treatment Procedure

- The operator provides a resistant force in the direction of hip flexion and knee extension.
- The rectus femoris muscle is isometrically contracted to optimum.
- During the postisometric relaxation phase, the hip is passively extended.
- Knee flexion is thereby increased, and starting from this new position the process is repeated, making sure, however, that hip extension is held to a minimum (Fig. **b**).

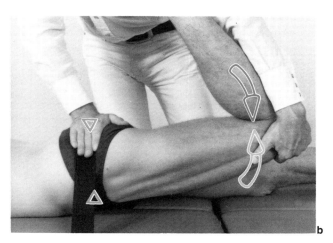

b

### Remarks

In an alternative procedure, the rectus femoris can be stretched directly over the knee joint, which, however, is often associated with pain resulting from pressure exerted to the femoropatellar joint.

# Adductor Longus Muscle, Adductor Brevis Muscle, Adductor Magnus Muscle, Gracilis Muscle

## NMT 2

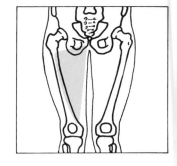

### Indication (Fig. a)

*Motion testing:* Leg abduction is diminished with soft endfeel.

*Pain:* The pain radiates toward the inguinal area at the medial side of the thigh. There is pain at the point of insertion of the muscle when palpated.

*Muscle testing:* The adductor muscles are shortened with typical pain when stretched.

### Positioning

- The patient lies on the nonvolved side.
- The leg close to the examination table is flexed assuring pelvis stabilization.
- The operator fixates the patient's pelvis with one hand.
- The other arm grasps the treatment leg, which has been extended both in the hip and knee joint.

*Note:* One should avoid contact in the area of the pes anserinus.

Passive abduction of the leg is introduced to stretch the leg maximally.

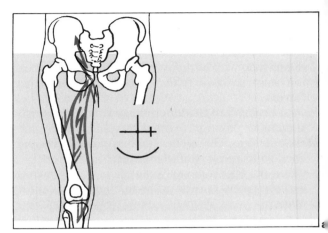

### Treatment Procedure

- The operator provides a resistant force against leg adduction.
- Optimal isometric contraction of the adductor muscles.
- During the postisometric relaxation phase, the leg is passively abducted (Fig. **b**). Starting from this new position, the procedure is repeated.

### Remarks

With this technique, the entire adductor muscle group is stretched.

When applying this technique with the knee joint flexed, gracilis muscle action is eliminated, and only the adductor muscles of the uniarticular joints are treated (Fig. **c**).

If there is medial knee instability, this technique may be difficult to perform and in many cases may even be contraindicated.

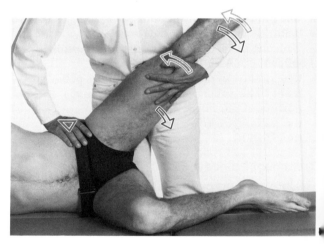

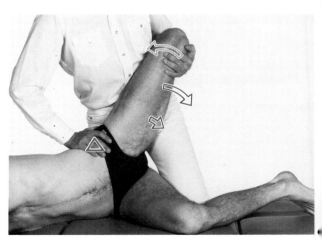

# Biceps Femoris Muscle, Semitendinosus Muscle, Semimembranosus Muscle

## NMT 2

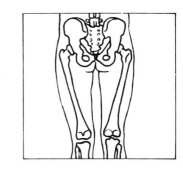

### Indication (Fig. a)

*Motion testing:* Hip flexion is diminished (with the knee extended), abrupt endfeel. (An abrupt reflexive barrier indicates a pathologic Lasègue sign.)
*Pain:* Chronic. Localized to the posterior thigh.
*Muscle testing:* The hamstring muscles are shortened with typical pain when stretched.

### Positioning

- The patient is supine.
  The nontreatment leg and the pelvis portion on that side are stabilized with a belt.
- With the patient's knee extended, passive hip flexion is introduced to the barrier.
- The operator supports the patient's lower leg and foot on his shoulder, while with his hands he assures knee extension and controls leg rotation.

### Treatment Procedure

- The operator's shoulder provides the resistant force.
  The hamstring muscles are isometrically contracted to optimum.
- During the postisometric relaxation phase, the muscles are passively stretched by increasing hip flexion.
- The process is repeated starting from the new position.

### Remarks

In the presence of a painful hip joint stretch should be effected utilizing the action of the Knee.

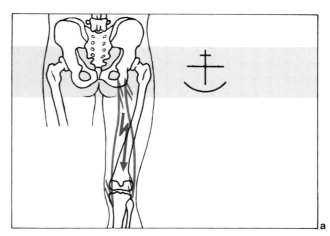

a

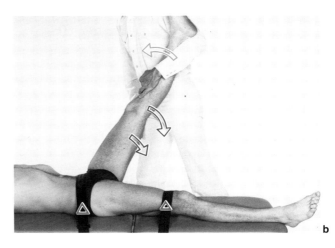

b

# Gastrocnemius and Soleus Muscles (Triceps Surae Muscle)

## NMT 2

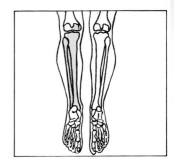

### Indication (Fig. a)

*Motion testing:* With the knee joint extended, there is diminished dorsiflexion joint with soft endfeel at the ankle.

*Pain:* There is pain in the patient's heel both when weight-bearing of during rest.

*Muscle testing:* The gastrocnemius and soleus muscles (triceps surae muscle) are shortened with typical pain when stretched.

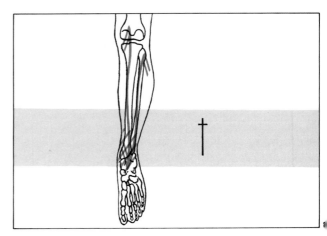

### Positioning

- The patient is supine and the treatment leg is flexed both at the hip and knee.
- The operator places one arm around the patient's thigh.
- The other hand is placed over the patient's calcaneus, introducing maximal dorsiflexion (Fig. **b**).

### Treatment Procedure

- The operator provides a resistant force to the calcaneus and forefoot.
- Optimal isometric contraction of the gastrocnemius and soleus muscle (Fig. **b**).
- During the postisometric relaxation phase, the knee is passively extended with the foot held in dorsiflexion (Fig. **c**).
- From this position the same procedure is repeated, and the mobility gain may be correlated with the stretch effected in the muscle.

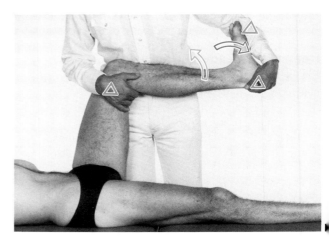

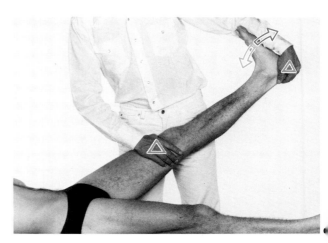

# Wrist Joint Extensors

## NMT 2

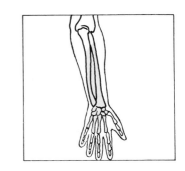

### Indication (Fig. a)

*Motion testing:* With the elbow extended, there is diminished wrist flexion (diminished finger flexion with wrist joint flexed); soft endfeel.
*Pain:* The extensor muscles are painful on palpation. Pain occurs at the end of the wrist flexion (finger flexion).
*Muscle testing:* The wrist joint extensors are shortened (finger extensor muscles) with typical pain when stretched.

### Positioning

- The patient is sitting with his elbow flexed approximately 90°.
- While the operator places one hand around the patient's elbow, he introduces with his other hand maximal passive wrist flexion (Fig. **b**).

### Treatment Procedure

- The operator provides a resistant force to the patient's hand (hand, fingers).
- Optimal isometric contraction of the wrist extensors.
- During the postisometric relaxation phase, passive extension of the elbow is introduced with wrist flexion maintained (Fig. **b**), leading to muscle stretch. Wrist flexion is increased, and starting from this new position, the procedure is repeated.

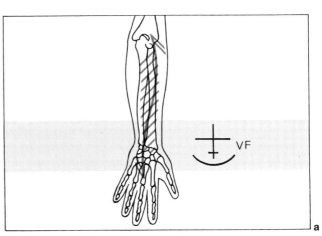

a

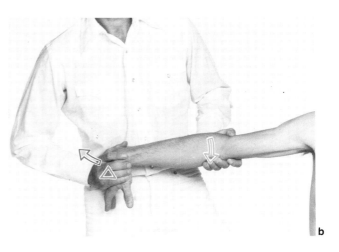

b

# Shoulder Joint

## Mobilization without Impulse: Traction

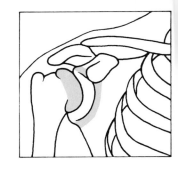

### Indication (Fig. a)

*Motion testing:* Shoulder motion restriction with hard endfeel. Diminished translatory motion with hard-elastic endfeel.

*Pain:* Acute or chronic. Pain is localized or may radiate to the lateral side of the patient's arm.
Pain with motion or, significantly, during rest.
Occasionally, the pain may only occur at the end of movement.

*Muscle testing:* The descending portion of the trapezius muscle and the pectoralis major muscle are often shortened while the medial shoulder fixator muscles may be weak.

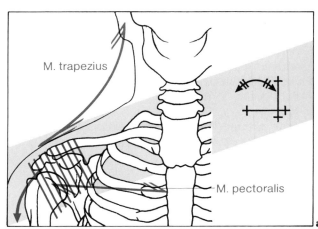

### Positioning

- Patient is supine and close to the edge of the examination table.
- The patient's shoulder and thorax are fixated with a belt.
- A second belt is wrapped around the operator's pelvis and patient's arm.
- The operator places one hand on the medial side of the patient's arm close to the joint and under the belt. The other hand is placed over the flexed elbow providing additional fixation.
- The present neutral position in the shoulder joint is found (Fig. **b**).

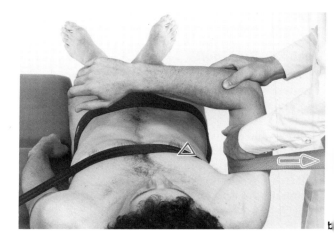

### Treatment Procedure

- Passive mobilization is introduced perpendicular to the treatment plane.
- One should avoid any angular motion (Fig. **b**).

### Remarks

This technique is well suited for pain treatment, but not beyond the application of traction II.
One should pay particular attention to the following: If the anterior portion of the capsule is irritated, hand placement close to the joint may cause pain. This may be prevented by placing the hand more distally.

# Shoulder Joint

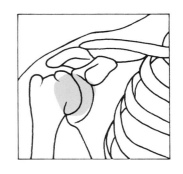

## Mobilization without Impulse: Inferior Direction

### Indication (Fig. a)

*Motion testing:* Shoulder abduction-elevation are restricted, as may be internal and external rotation with hard endfeel. Diminished inferior translatory motion with hard-elastic endfeel.

*Pain:* Acute or chronic pain.

Localized or radiating to the lateral side of the arm. Pain occurs both with motion or even more significantly during rest.

The pain may occasionally occur at the end of range of motion only.

### Positioning

– Patient is supine and close to the edge of the examination table.
– The shoulder is fixated with a belt or a fixation bar.
– The operator places both hands over the arm distal to the shoulder joint but proximal to the elbow joint (Fig. **b**).
– The present neutral position of the shoulder joint is determined.

### Treatment Procedure

Passive inferior mobilization is effected parallel to the plane of treatment (Fig. **b**).

### Remarks

Unless inferior translatory motion is normal, full angular motion in the shoulder joint is impossible.

Thus, if angular mobility is diminished, this mobilization technique is in most cases of central importance.

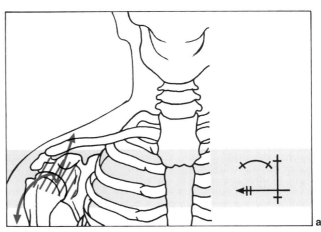

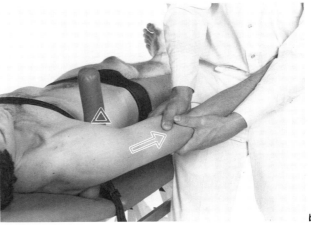

# Shoulder Joint

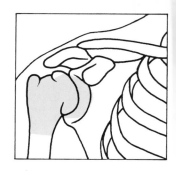

## Mobilization without Impulse: Posterior Direction

### Indication (Fig. a)

*Motion testing:* Internal rotation or elevation restriction with hard endfeel. Diminished posterior translatory motion with hard endfeel.

*Pain:* Acute or chronic.
Anterior capsule components are frequently painful on pressure.

*Pain:* Pain occurs both with motion and with rest.

*Muscle testing:* The pectoralis major and the descending portion of the trapezius muscles are often shortened, whereas the medial shoulder fixator muscles are often weak.

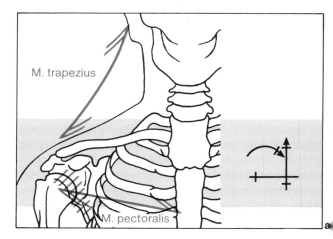

### Positioning

- The patient is supine and close to the edge of the examination table.
- The shoulder blade is supported with a sandbag or wedge.
- The operator grasps with one hand the patient's flexed elbow, stablizing the entire arm against his body.
- The present neutral position of the shoulder joint is found.
- The operator's other hand is placed flat over the anterior portion of the patient's arm proximal to the joint (Fig. **b**).

### Treatment Procedure

- Traction level I, which is maintained throughout the treatment.
- Passive posterior mobilization parallel to the treatment plane (Fig. **b**).

### Remarks

Additional angular motion components should not be included.

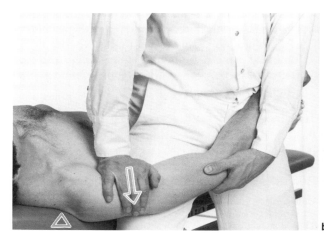

# Shoulder Joint

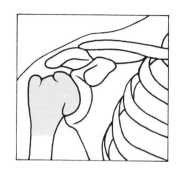

## Mobilization without Impulse: Anterior Direction

### Indication (Fig. a)

*Motion testing:* External rotation or extension restriction with hard endfeel.

Diminished anterior translatory motion with hard endfeel.

*Pain:* Chronic or localized.

The anterior capsule components are tender on pressure.

Pain occurs with motion but may be significant at rest.

*Muscle testing:* Often the descending portion of the trapezius and the pectoralis major muscles are shortened, whereas the medial shoulder fixator muscles are weak.

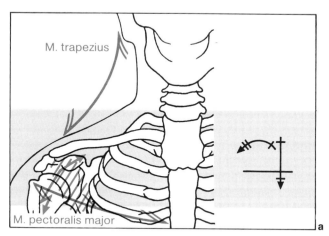

### Positioning

- The patient is prone and close to the edge of the examination table.
- A sandbag or wedge is placed under the patient's coracoid process, which provides certain stabilization of the shoulder blade.
- The operator places one hand over the distal portion of the patient's arm.
- The present neutral position is found.
- Often the arm is in the same plane as the spine of the scapula.
- The operator places his other hand over the posterior side of the patient's arm close to the joint (Fig. **b**).

*Note:* One should make sure that the coracoid is supported on the anterior side only. The head of the humerus, which will undergo anterior mobilization, should not be supported. If the anterior support is not sufficient to stablize the shoulder blade, a belt may be utilized in addition.

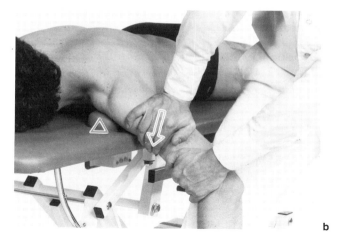

### Treatment Procedure

- Traction level I is maintained throughout the entire treatment procedure.
- Passive anterior mobilization parallel to the treatment plane (Fig. **b**).

### Remarks

One must avoid additional angular motion components.
If there is pain with this procedure, one should reevaluate the patient's position and reexamine the present neutral position.

# Sternoclavicular Joint

## Mobilization without Impulse: Posterior (Inferior) Direction

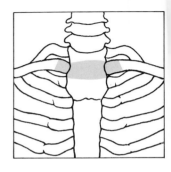

### Indication (Fig. a)

*Motion testing:* Diminished posterior (or inferior) translatory motion with hard endfeel.

*Pain:* Pain with movement. The joint capsule is tender on palpation.

*Muscle testing:* The sternocleidomastoid and scalene muscles may be shortened.

### Positioning

- The patient is supine.
- For posterior mobilization: the operator places the pisiform bone of one hand over the medial end of the clavicle. The other hand supports the mobilizing hand.
  (For inferior mobilization: the medial clavicle is fixated superiorly with the operator's thumb and index finger.)

### Treatment Procedure

- Posterior mobilization of the medial clavicle portion (or inferior).

*Note:* The posterior mobilization procedure can be carried out synchronously with the patient's exhalation. The pressure applied to the area around the joint capsule should be minimal.

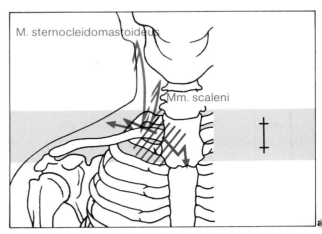

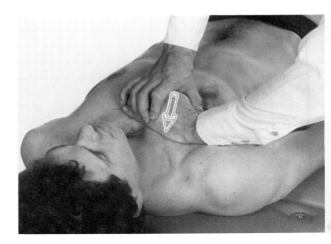

# Acromioclavicular Joint

## NMT 1, Superior Direction

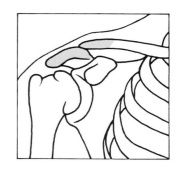

### Indication (Fig. a)

*Motion testing:* Diminished anteroinferior translatory motion of the clavicle. Abduction of the arm is restricted and painful.

*Pain:* The pain is chronic, localized and exacerbated when provoked.

The joint cavity is tender on palpation.

Abduction movement of the arm may occasionally cause pain.

*Muscle testing:* The descending portion of the trapezius muscle may be shortened.

### Positioning

– The patient is sitting upright with the thoracic spine extended.
– The operator stands behind the patient and fixates the patient's clavicle with the palmar side of his forearm.
– With his other hand, he fixates the patient's head, providing stabilization to the cervical spine (Fig. **b**).

### Treatment Procedure

– Active mobilization is effected by lifting the patient's shoulder blade against the fixated clavicle.
– The mobilization procedure is performed while the patient inhales (Fig. **b**).

### Remarks

In this maneuver, the acromion undergoes a superior translatory motion in relation to the clavicle.

If with this maneuver pain becomes prominent in the cervical spine, the procedure must be terminated. One should then examine and, if necessary, treat the cervical spine.

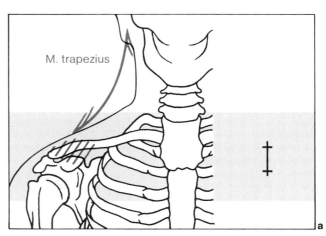

M. trapezius

a

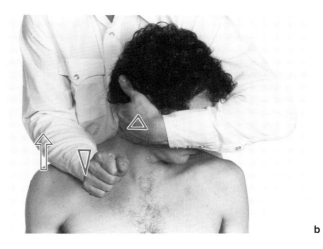

b

# Shoulder Blade

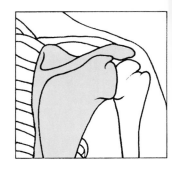

## Mobilization without Impulse: Superior or Inferior, Medial or Lateral Direction

### Indication (Fig. a)

*Motion testing:* Restricted subscapular gliding motion of the shoulder blade.

Often shoulder joint motion is restricted as well.

*Pain:* Diffuse, subscapular and interscapular.

### Positioning

- Patient is in the side-lying position with his hip and knees flexed. The thoracic spine is slightly flexed and stabilized.
- The operator, standing in front of the patient, places the fingertips of one hand over the inferior angle of the shoulder blade while the other hand is placed flat over the spine of the scapula (Fig. **b**).

### Treatment Procedure

- Passive superoinferior and mediolateral mobilization of the shoulder blade (Fig. **b**).

### Remarks

Quite frequently the shoulder blade fixator muscles undergo reflexive contraction, precluding the hand placement described above. In the event of reflexive contractions, the operator places one hand broadly, in a vicelike manner, over the inferior angle and then pushes the shoulder blade over his hand.

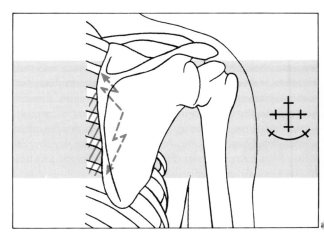

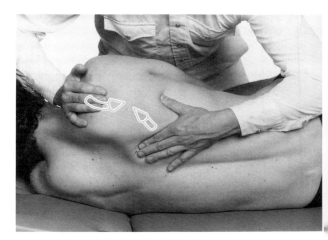

# Elbow Joint

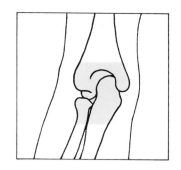

## Mobilization without Impulse: Traction

### Indication (Fig a)

*Motion testing:* Angular flexion or extension restriction with hard endfeel.
Diminished translatory motion with hard endfeel.
*Pain:* Chronic and localized. Pain on movement or with loading force application.
*Muscle testing:* The biceps brachii or the wrist extensors may be shortened, and the triceps brachii muscle can be weak.

### Positioning

- Patient is supine.
- The patient's arm is fixated with a belt in such a manner that the olecranon rests beyond the edge of the examination table.
- The present neutral position is found.
- The operator grasps with one hand the patient's wrist and stabilizes the patient's forearm against his body. The other hand is placed broadly over the patient's forearm proximal to the joint (Fig. **b**).

### Treatment Procedure

- Traction is introduced perpendicular to the treatment plane, i.e., at right angle to the forearm's axis.
- Avoid any other angular motion component.

### Remarks

Traction in the elbow joint is quite small because the collateral ligaments are taut and strong.

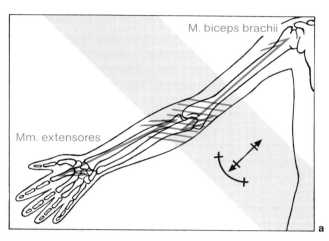

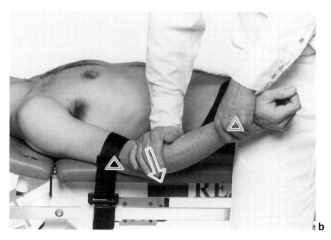

# Elbow Joint

## Mobilization without Impulse: Traction

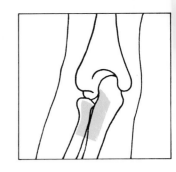

### Indication (Fig. a)

*Motion testing:* Diminished angular pronation or supination motion with hard endfeel.
Diminished translatory motion with hard endfeel.

*Pain:* Chronic and localized. The humeroradial joint space is tender on palpation, as may be the annular ligament of the radius.
Pain may occur both during rest and with movement.

*Muscle testing:* The extensors of the wrist and the fingers may be shortened.

### Positioning

- Patient is supine.
- The operator fixates, with one hand, the patient's arm proximal to the joint.
- The other hand is placed in a vicelike manner over the distal end of the radius (Fig. **b**).
- The present neutral position of the joint is found.

### Treatment Procedure

- Traction is effected along the axis of the radius (Fig. **b**).

*Note:* One should avoid any other angular motion component. Traction in the radiohumeral joint is always accompanied by joint gliding in the radioulnar joint.

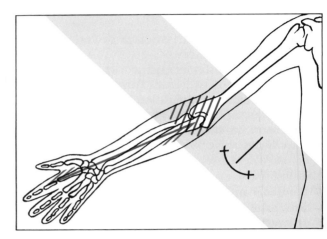

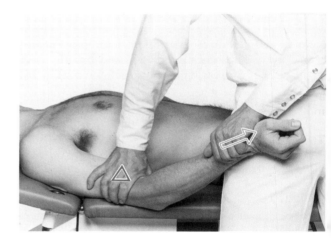

# Proximal Radioulnar Joint

## Mobilization without Impulse: Posterior-Cubital Direction

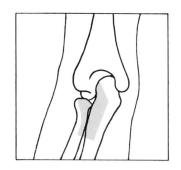

### Indication (Fig. a)

*Motion testing:* Angular pronation and supination restriction with hard endfeel.
Diminished posterior or anterior translatory motion with hard endfeel.
*Pain:* Chronic and localized. The humeroradial joint space is tender on palpation. Pain may occur both with motion and during rest.
*Muscle testing:* The wrist extensor and finger extensor muscles may be shortened.

### Positioning

- Patient is sitting, with his forearm resting on the examination table.
- The present neutral position of the joint is found.
- The operator fixates the patient's ulna with one hand.
  The thenar eminence of the other hand makes contact with the radial head (Fig. **b**).

*Note:* For posterior mobilization the operator stands at the medial side of the arm, whereas for anterior mobilization, he stands at the lateral side of the arm.

### Treatment Procedure

- Gliding motion is introduced in the posterior (or cubital) direction.

### Remarks

The operator should make sure that his hand is placed gently around the patient's elbow in order to avoid possible pain especially if insertion tendinopathies are present.
Radioulnar mobilization is always accompanied by mobilization in the radiohumeral joint.

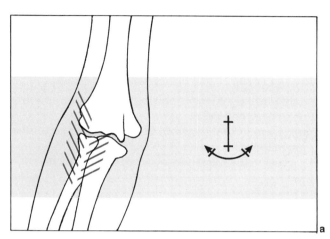

a

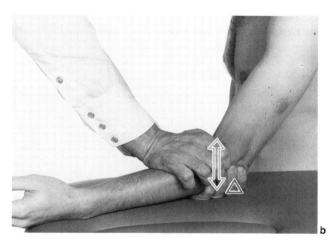

b

# Distal Radioulnar Joint

## Mobilization without Impulse: Posterior-Cubital Direction

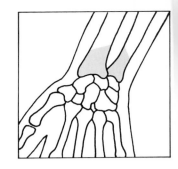

### Indication (Fig. a)

*Motion testing:* Pronation and supination motion restriction with hard endfeel. Angular motion restriction with hard endfeel in the wrist may occur occasionally.

Diminished posteroanterior translatory motion with hard endfeel.

*Pain:* Chronic and localized. The joint space is tender on palpation.

Occasionally, pain may occur with movement.

### Positioning

– The patient is sitting, with his forearm resting in the supinated position on the examination table. The operator fixates the ulna distally in a gentle manner (Fig. **b**).
– The operator places the other hand distally over the radius, also gently (Fig. **b**).

### Treatment Procedure

– Passive posterior or cubital mobilization of the radius (Fig. **b**).

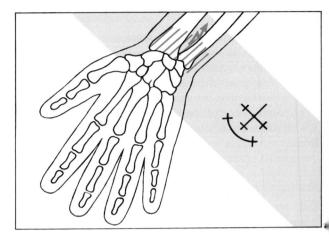

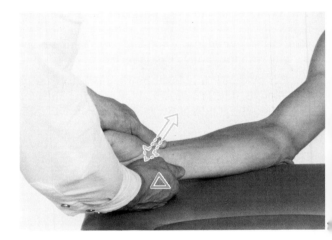

# Proximal (Distal) Wrist Joint

## Mobilization without Impulse: Traction

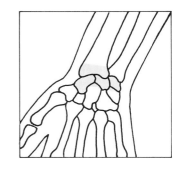

### Indication (Fig. a)

*Motion testing:* Angular motion restriction in at least one plane of the wrist with hard endfeel.
Diminished translatory motion with hard endfeel.

*Pain:* Chronic and localized. Pain is associated with movement and occasionally may occur only toward the end of the range of motion.

### Positioning

- The patient is sitting.
- If traction is intended for the proximal wrist joint, the patient's forearm is fixated proximally.
- If traction is intended for the distal wrist joint portion, the proximal carpal row is fixated as well.
- The operator places his other hand in a vicelike manner over the proximal and distal wrist bones, respectively.
- The present neutral position is found (Fig. **b**).

### Treatment Procedure

- Traction to the wrist joint is introduced, whereby the operator holds the forearm of the fixating hand toward his trunk and moves the forearm of his mobilizing hand in the direction of traction (Fig. **b**).

### Remarks

This technique is particularly well suited for pain treatment, but one should be careful not to exceed traction level II.
Additional angular motion components must be avoided.

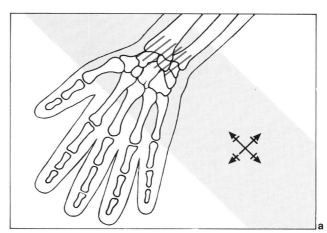

a

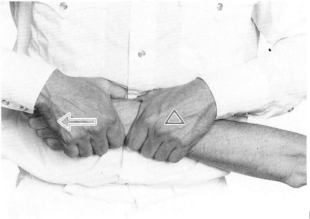

b

# Proximal (Distal) Wrist Joint

## Mobilization without Impulse: Palmar (Dorsal) Direction

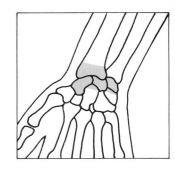

### Indication (Fig. a)

*Motion testing:* Angular motion restriction of wrist flexion and/or extension with hard endfeel.
Diminished translatory wrist extension and flexion motion with hard endfeel.

*Pain:* Pain occurs toward the end of range of motion.

### Positioning

- The patient is sitting.
- The patient's forearm rests on the examination table. The operator fixates the patient's forearm proximal to the joint.
- The operator places his other hand in the following manner:
  - Over the proximal carpal bones for mobilization of the proximal wrist joint.
  - Over the distal carpal bones for mobilization of the distal wrist joint.
- The present neutral position is found (Fig. **b**).

*Note:* It is important to be as close to the joint as possible.

### Treatment Procedure

- Traction level 1.
- Wrist flexion or extension mobilization in the proximal or distal wrist joint, respectively (Fig. **b**).

### Remarks

If pain appears with this mobilization, it is recommended that the joint first be treated with traction only.

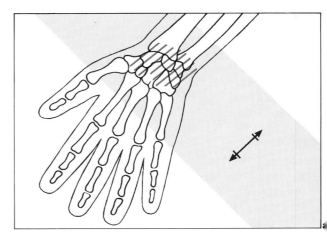

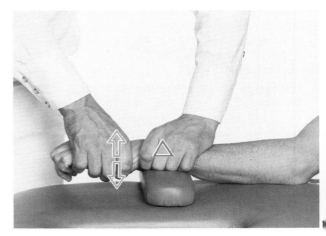

# Proximal Wrist Joint

## Mobilization without Impulse: Ulnar (Radial) Direction

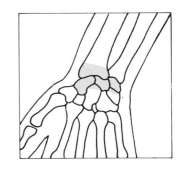

### Indication (Fig. a)

*Motion testing:* Diminished angular radius or ulnar abduction with hard endfeel.
Restricted translatory movement in the direction of the ulna (radius) with hard endfeel.
*Pain:* Pain appears at the end of the range of movement.

### Positioning

- Patient is sitting.
- The patient's arm rests with the ulnar or the radial side on the examination table.
- The operator fixates with one hand the patient's forearm proximal to the joint.
- He places his other hand gently over the proximal row of the carpal bones.
- The present neutral position is found (Fig. **b**).

### Treatment Procedure

- Traction level I
- Passive mobilization in the direction of the ulna (Fig. **b**) or radius.

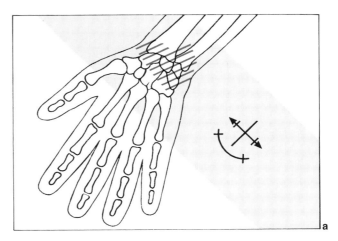

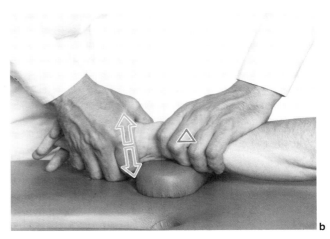

# Carpal Bones

## Mobilization without Impulse: Dorsal (Palmar) Direction

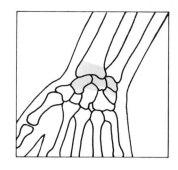

### Indication (Fig. a)

*Motion Testing:* Diminished dorsal extension, palmar flexion and/or radius and ulnar abduction. Restricted translatory movement of wrist in the dorsal or palmar direction with hard endfeel.

*Pain:* Acute or chronic; localized.

Pain appears at the end of the range of movement.

### Positioning

– Patient is sitting.
– The operator braces the forearm of the patient against his (the operator's) body, fixates with thumb and index finger of one hand the appropriate bone in the proximal row of carpal bones.
– With thumb and index finger of the other hand the operator fixates the articulating distal carpal bone.
– The intracarpal joint is in the present neutral position.

### Treatment Procedure

– Traction Level I
– Mobilization of the distal carpal bone in the dorsal (palmar) direction.

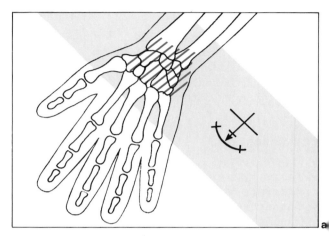

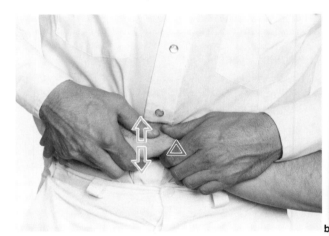

# Finger Joints

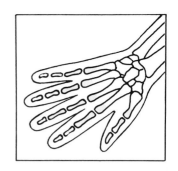

## Mobilization without Impulse: Traction

### Indication (Fig. a)

*Motion testing:* Angular flexion or extension motion restriction with hard endfeel. Diminished translatory motion with hard endfeel.
*Pain:* Acute or chronic; localized.
  Pain may occur with movement or during rest.

### Positioning

- Patient is sitting.
- The operator stabilizes the patient's forearm by placing it against his body. He fixates the restricted joint by placing his thumb and index finger of one hand proximal to the joint, while the thumb and index finger of the other hand are placed distal to the restricted joint.
- The present neutral position is found (Fig. **b**).

*Note:* Hand placement should be gentle and as close to the joint as possible.

### Treatment Procedure

- Passive traction, perpendicular to the treatment plane (Fig. **b**).

### Remarks

This technique is well suited for pain treatment, but one should not go beyond traction level 2.

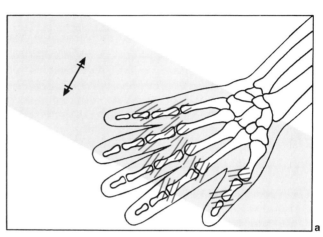

a

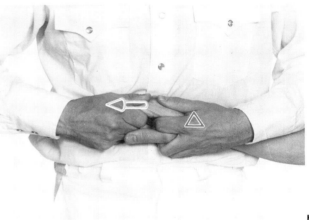

b

# Finger Joints

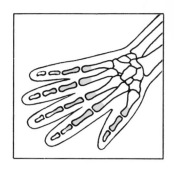

## Mobilization without Impulse: Palmar (Dorsal) Direction

### Indication (Fig. a)

*Motion testing:* Flexion (extension) restriction with hard endfeel.
Diminished translatory palmar (or dorsal) motion with hard endfeel.

*Pain:* Chronic and localized. Pain may occur with movement or during rest.

*Muscle testing:* The finger extensor muscles may be shortened.

### Positioning

– Patient is sitting with the forearm resting on the examination table.
– The operator fixates the patient's restricted joint proximal to the joint space.
– He then places his thenar eminence and index finger of the other hand distal to the joint space (Fig. **b**).
– The present neutral position is found.

### Treatment Procedure

– Traction level 1.
– Passive mobilization in the palmar (dorsal) direction, parallel to the treatment plane.

*Note:* The carpometacarpal joint is treated accordingly, i.e., depending on whether flexion or extension restriction is present.

Thus, diminished flexion motion is treated with mobilization in the ulnar direction, and diminished extension with mobilization in the radial direction.

If there is diminished abduction, dorsal mobilization should be utilized, whereas in case of diminished adduction mobilization is in the palmar direction.

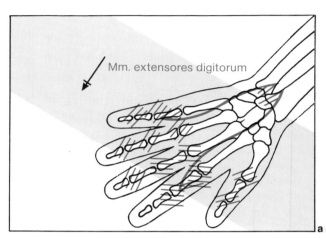

Mm. extensores digitorum

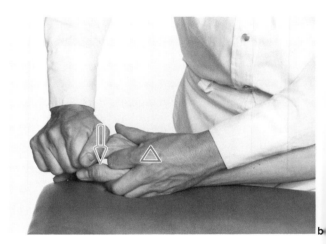

# Hip Joint

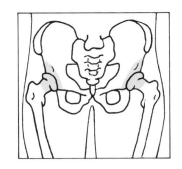

## Mobilization without Impulse: Traction (Inferior)

### Indication (Fig. a)

*Motion testing:* Angular motion restriction with hard endfeel. Restricted inferior translatory motion with hard endfeel.

*Pain:* Pain may be localized or radiate toward the symphysis pubis as well as the lateral thigh. May be chronic or acute. Pain may be found both at rest and with movement, and may occur when movement is initiated.

Pain at the end of flexion or internal rotation movement.

*Muscle testing:* Often, the rectus femoris, piriformis, and iliopsoas muscles are shortened. The gluteal muscles are often weak. The hamstring muscles and tensor fasciae latae muscle are frequently weak as well.

### Positioning

- Patient is supine.
- The pelvis is fixated with a belt or a stationary bar.
- The operator places both hands flat over the malleoli with the patient's knee extended.
- The joint is brought to its present neutral positione.

*Note:* Since the femoral head receives some of its arterial supply through the ligament of the capital head, traction level 3 should not be applied for longer than 10–15 seconds.

The operator must place his hands proximal to the ankle joint. It is imperative that the joint be positioned exactly in the present neutral position, requiring that the patient be totally relaxed and pain free (Fig. **b**).

### Treatment Procedures

- Traction is along the leg's axis.

### Remarks

- If pain appears with the mobilization procedure, one should reevaluate the present neutral position.
- If there is a disease process affecting the knee joint, this treatment technique may be difficult to apply or may actually be contraindicated.

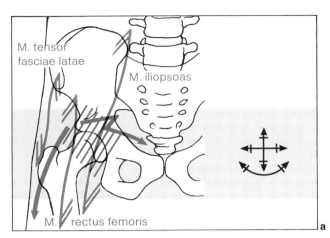

M. tensor fasciae latae

M. iliopsoas

M. rectus femoris

a

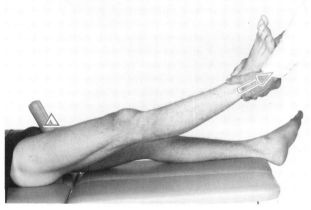

b

# Hip Joint

## Mobilization without Impulse: Posterior Direction

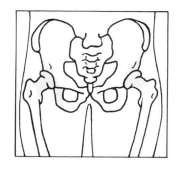

### Indication (Fig. a)

*Motion testing:* Angular flexion restriction with hard endfeel. Diminished posterior translatory motion with hard endfeel.

*Pain:* Chronic and localized. Pain with loading force application or when movement is initiated.

*Muscle testing:* Frequently, the iliopsoas and rectus femoris muscles are shortened with the gluteus maximus, medius, and abdominal muscles being weak.

### Positioning

- The patient is supine and resting close to the edge of the examination table.
- The noninvolved leg is flexed maximally at the hip and knee joint and held in this position by the patient. This also reverses the lumbar lordosis.
- The affected leg is brought to its present neutral position.
- The operator utilizes a belt to counteract the leg's weight.
- The fixating hand is placed between the posterior side of the thigh and belt, allowing a soft grip and longitudinal traction (Fig. **b**).

### Treatment Procedure

- Passive posterior mobilization.

*Note:* Attention is to be paid to having the mobilizing hand as close to the joint as possible and to moving the entire thigh in a parallel fashion, that is, there should be no angular compression.

### Remarks

This technique is physically demanding for the operator, and if the treatment procedure is to be carried out over a longer period of time, one should employ special tables and aids.

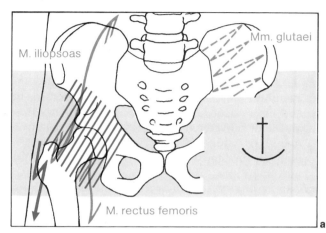

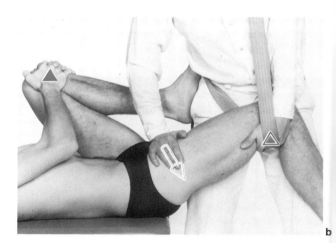

# Hip Joint

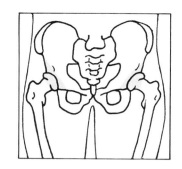

## Mobilization without Impulse: Anterior Direction

### Indication (Fig. a)

*Motion testing:* Angular extension restriction.
Diminished anterior translatory motion with hard endfeel.
*Pain:* Chronic and localized, may be present with loading or when motion is initiated.
*Muscle testing:* In most instances, the iliopsoas and rectus femoris muscles are shortened and the gluteus maximus and gluteus medius muscles are weak.

### Positioning

– The patient is prone with both legs hanging beyond the table, but the pelvis resting securely on the table. The hip and knee joints are slightly flexed and the feet make contact with the floor.
– The operator stands on the involved side.
– A belt that is placed over the operator's shoulder is used to hold the patient's thigh.
– The operator places one hand on the patient's leg and introduces 90° flexion to the knee while stabilizing the patient's leg with his own leg.
– The joint is brought to its present neutral position. The operator places his other hand flat and close to the joint over the patient's thigh.

### Treatment Procedure

– Passive anterior mobilization.
– While performing the treatment procedure, the operator bends his knees slightly in order to "move" the entire leg in an anterior direction, which prevent any angular motion from taking place.

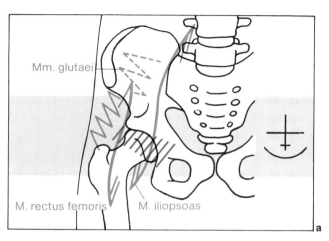

Mm. glutaei

M. rectus femoris    M. iliopsoas

a

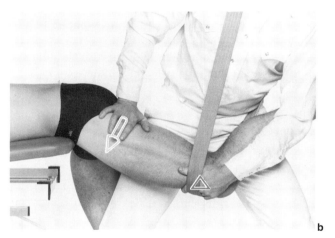

b

# Hip Joint

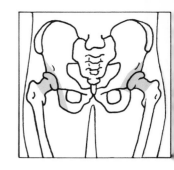

## Mobilization without Impulse: Lateral Traction

### Indication (Fig. a)

*Motion testing:* Angular motion restriction in all planes with hard elastic endfeel. Diminished lateral translatory motion with hard endfeel.

*Pain:* Acute or chronic. Localized or radiating to the inguinal region, the lateral or medial thigh. Pain with initiation of movement.

*Muscle testing:* In the majority of cases, the tensor fasciae latae, piriformis, or adductor muscles are shortened, whereas the gluteal muscles are weak.

### Positioning

- The patient is supine.
- The hip joint is brought to the present neutral position.
- Using a belt, the pelvis is fixated and thus prevented from moving laterally.
- The treatment hand is placed close to the joint on the medial side of the patient's thigh.
- A second belt may be placed over the operator's hand and pelvis in order to facilitate mobilization.

### Treatment Procedure

- Passive lateral mobilization.

*Note:* With this procedure, it is important that the operator's nontreatment hand (stabilization hand) is placed distally following along with the lateral movement.

This technique is particularly useful for treatment of pain.

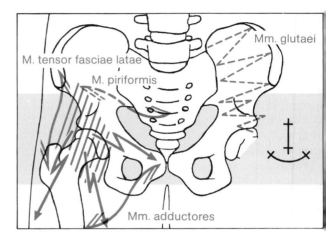

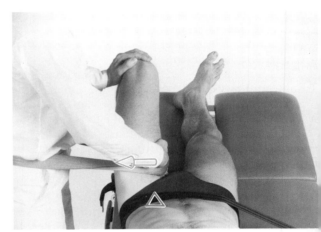

# Femoropatellar Gliding

## Mobilization without Impulse: Distal (Medial/Lateral) Direction

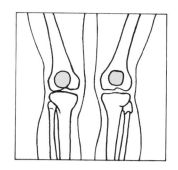

### Indication (Fig. a)

*Motion testing:* Diminished joint gliding of the patella associated with decreased knee joint extension and flexion.

*Pain:* Pain is chronic and retropatellar. Pain gets worse with loading (weight-bearing) and increasing knee flexion.

*Muscle testing:* The rectus femoris and tensor fasciae latae muscles are shortened and the vastus medialis muscle is weak.

### Positioning

- Patient is supine.
- The knee is slightly flexed and supported by a sandbag.
- With his forearm resting on the patient's thigh, the operator places the hand flat over the patient's patella.
- The other hand is used for support (Fig. **b**).

### Treatment Procedure

- Passive distal mobilization of the patella (medial and lateral) (Fig. **b**).

*Note:* One should provide minimal retropatellar compression with this mobilization technique.

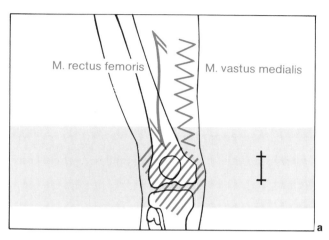

M. rectus femoris    M. vastus medialis

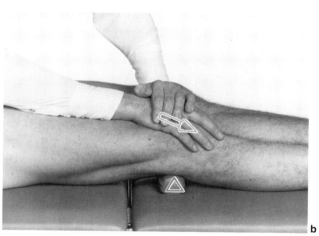

# Knee Joint

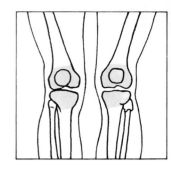

## Mobilization without Impulse: Traction

### Indication (Fig. a)

*Motion testing:* Angular flexion or extension restriction with hard endfeel.
  Optional: Diminished translatory motion with hard endfeel.
*Pain:* Localized and subacute. Pain occurs both with movement and during rest.
*Muscle testing:* The rectus femoris muscle is shortened, as may be the tensor fasciae latae and hamstring muscles. The vastus medialis muscle is weak.

### Positioning

– The patient is prone, and his thigh is fixated with a belt.
– The operator places both hands gently over the patient's malleoli (Fig. **b**).
– The present neutral position is found.

### Treatment Procedure

– Traction is applied by pulling on the patient's lower leg along its axis (Fig. **b**).

### Remarks

This technique is particularly well suited for treating pain but with the force not beyond traction level 2.

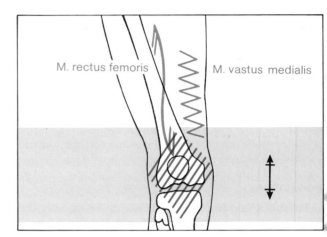

M. rectus femoris     M. vastus medialis

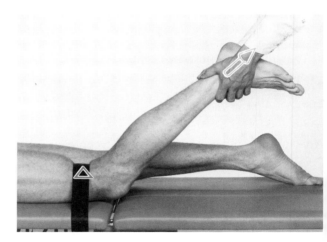

# Knee Joint

## Mobilization without Impulse: Anterior (Posterior) Direction

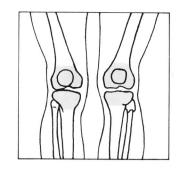

### Indication (Fig. a)

*Motion testing:* Angular extension (flexion) restriction with hard endfeel.
   Diminished anterior translatory motion with hard endfeel.
*Pain:* Pain is chronic and localized. May occur both with movement and at rest.
*Muscle testing:* The rectus femoris muscle and sometimes the tensor fasciae latae and hamstring muscles are shortened. The vastus medialis muscle is weak.

### Positioning

– Patient is prone (or supine).
– The patient's leg is beyond the end of the treatment table.
– The operator places one hand over the distal end of the restricted leg while he places his other hand proximally and flat on the patient's leg (Figs. **b, c**).
– The present neutral position is found.

### Treatment Procedure

– Traction level 1
   – Passive anterior mobilization (Fig. **b**) and dorsal mobilization (Fig. **c**).

### Remarks

There should be no angular component. The neutral position may change with the treatment, requiring repositioning.
*Caveat:* If the knee joint is damaged, and in particular with cruciate ligament damage, one may use this technique, if at all, with careful force application only.

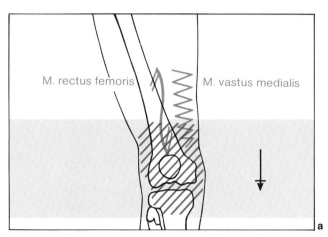

M. rectus femoris    M. vastus medialis

a

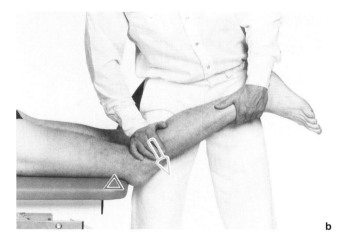

b

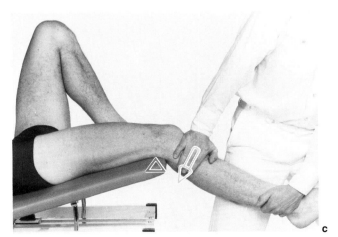

c

# Proximal (Distal) Tibiofibular Joint

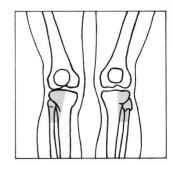

## Mobilization without Impulse: Anterior/Posterior Direction

### Indication (Fig. a)

*Motion testing:* Diminished anterior (or posterior) translatory motion with hard endfeel.

*Pain:* Lateral knee pain.

There is pain at the end of movement when the joint is brought to its maximal supination.

*Muscle testing:* The biceps femoris is shortened.

### Positioning

– The patient stands at the side of the table, resting his leg on the examination table.
– The operator places his thenar eminence flat over the fibular head supported by the other hand.

*Note:* If the operator performs posterior mobilization, the patient should be supine with the hip and knee joints slightly flexed.

### Treatment Procedure

– Passive anterior (or posterior) mobilization (Fig. **b**).

### Remarks

Lateral knee pain is often present when the proximal tibiofibular joint is affected.

It is important that the operator places his hands over the affected area in a gentle manner in order to prevent pain or fibular nerve compression.

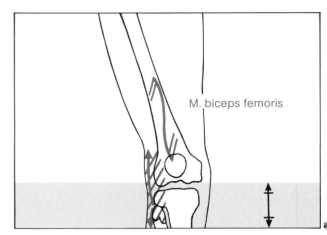

M. biceps femoris

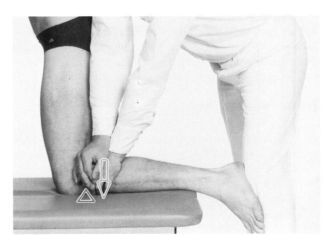

# Ankle (Talocrural) Joint

## Mobilization without Impulse: Traction

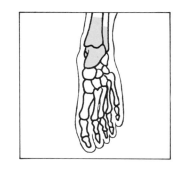

### Indication (Fig. a)

*Motion testing:* Angular dorsiflexion or plantar flex-
ion restriction with hard endfeel.
   Diminished translatory motion with hard endfeel.
*Pain:* Pain is either acute or chronic and localized.
   Pain occurs toward the end of movement.
*Muscle testing:* The gastrocnemius muscle may be
shortened.

### Positioning

– The patient is supine, with his foot beyond the
  examination table.
– The leg on the effected side is fixated with a belt.
– The operator grasps the patient's foot in a broad
  manner (vicelike) and as close to the joint as
  possible.
– The present neutral position is found.

### Treatment Procedure

– Traction along the axis of the leg (Fig. **b**).

### Remarks

This technique is especially well suited for treating pain, but the
force of traction should be carefully applied (not grater than
traction level 2).

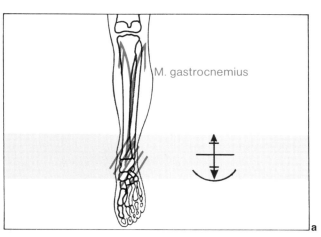

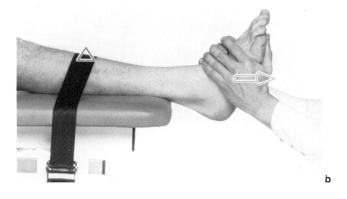

# Ankle (Talocrural) Joint

## Mobilization without Impulse: Anterior (Posterior) Direction

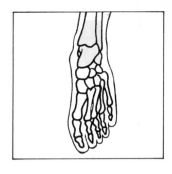

### Indication (Fig. a)

*Motion testing:* Angular plantar flexion (or dorsiflexion) restriction with hard endfeel. Diminished anterior (posterior) translatory motion with hard endfeel.

*Pain:* Chronic and localized. Pain at the end of movement.

*Muscle testing:* The gastrocnemius and soleus muscles may be shortened.

### Positioning

- The patient is prone (or supine) with his foot beyond the treatment table.
- In the prone position, the malleoli are supported with a sandbag.
- The operator grasps with one hand the patient's talus in a vicelike manner while his other hand grasps the patient's forefoot effecting additional fixation (Figs. **b, c**).
- The present neutral position is found.

### Treatment Procedure

- Traction level 1.
- Passive mobilization of the talus anteriorly (Fig. **b**) or posteriorly (Fig. **c**).

### Remarks

One should avoid any angular component.

*Caveat:* In situations in which there is significant tendon damage of this joint, one should be very careful to apply this technique, and in such a way as to avoid overstretch of the tendons.

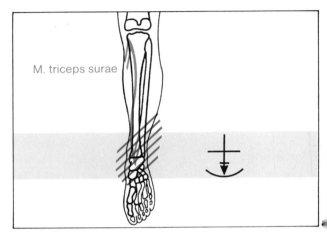

M. triceps surae

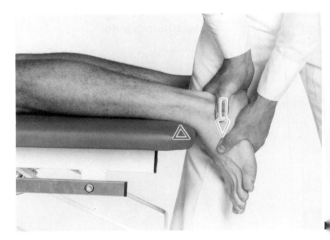

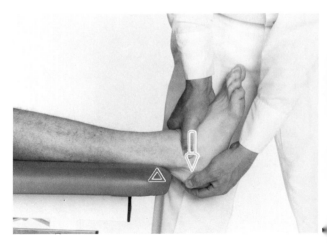

# Joints at the Hindfoot
# (Tarsal and Tarsometatarsal Joints)

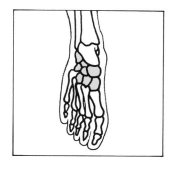

## Mobilization without Impulse: Plantar (Posterior) Direction

### Indication (Fig. a)

*Motion testing:* Diminished dorsal (or plantar) translatory motion with hard endfeel.
*Pain:* Static foot pain, acute or chronic and localized.
*Muscle testing:* The inferior set muscles are often weak.

### Positioning

- The patient is supine (or prone).
- The restricted joint is fixated proximally by the operator's hand.
- The operator places his other hand over the incriminated, restricted bones.

### Treatment Procedure

- Traction level 1
- Passive plantar (dorsal) mobilization, parallel to the plane of treatment (Fig. **b**).

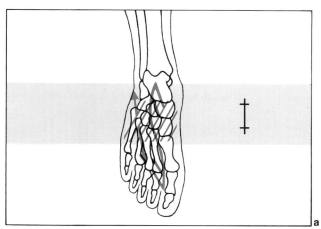

a

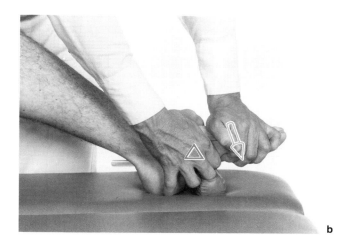

b

# Toe Joints

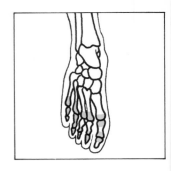

## Mobilization without Impulse: Traction

### Indication (Fig. a)

*Motion testing:* Angular flexion (extension) restriction with hard endfeel.
   Diminished translatory motion with hard endfeel.
*Pain:* Acute or chronic and localized. Pain appears with weight-bearing.

### Positioning

– The patient is supine.
– The operator places one hand proximal to the restricted joint (fixation) and the thumb and index finger of the other hand distal to the affected joint.
– The present neutral position is found (Fig. **b**).

### Treatment Procedure

– Traction perpendicular to the plane of treatment is introduced (Fig. **b**).

### Remarks

A soft, nonforceful grip is to be applied.

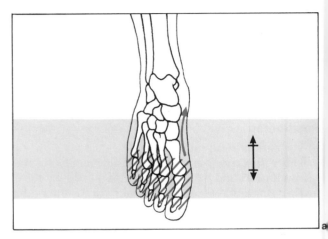

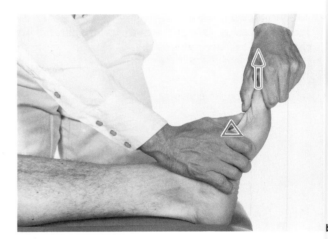

# Toe Joints

## Mobilization without Impulse: Plantar-Dorsal

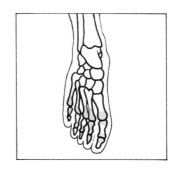

### Indication (Fig. a)

*Motion testing:* Restricted angular flexion ar extension, hard endfeel.
Diminished plantar or dorsal translatory motion
with hard endfeel.

*Pain:* Chronic and localized. Pain occurs when loading force is applied (weight-bearing).

### Positioning

– Patient is supine or prone.
– The operator places one hand proximally and the
other hand distally to the restricted joint (Fig. **b**).
– The present neutral position is found.

### Treatment Procedure

– Traction level 1.
Passive plantar or dorsal mobilization, which is
parallel to the treatment plane of the foot (Fig. **b**).

### Remarks

One should apply a gentle grip.

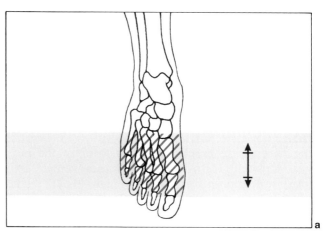

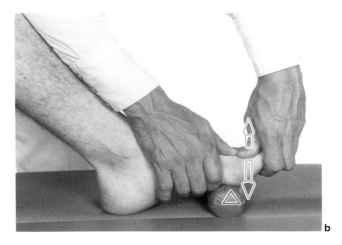

# 6    Home Exercise Training

In the majority of cases, manipulative therapy alone is not sufficient to bring about lasting improvement or even disappearance of a patient's symptoms. Thus, it is important that the patient learn a specific home training program that contains mobilizing, muscle stretching, and muscle strengthening components. As a rule, the exercises are introduced using the NMT 1 treatment procedures. They are of limited value, however, for a generalized program because the purpose of these exercises is to make the individual patient learn which specific movement patterns are appropriate for him. The NMT 2 and isometric strengthening exercises are presented in the following program.

To assure proper performance, the following points are important to remember:

- The selection of the specific, essential exercises
- The individual home training program should consist of no more than a total of five exercise parts
- Repeated evaluation is necessary to assure correct execution of the home exercise program
- Patient motivation can be significantly improved if the program is explained in an objective manner.

Frequently, manipulative therapy and the home exercises are supplemented by such considerations as:

- Dietary awareness
- General fitness
- Improvement of the workplace conditions
- Change in leisure and athletic activities

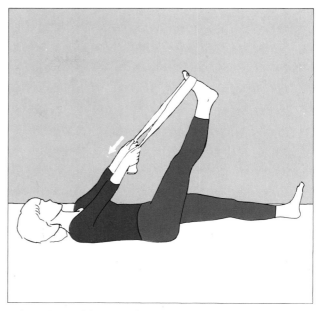

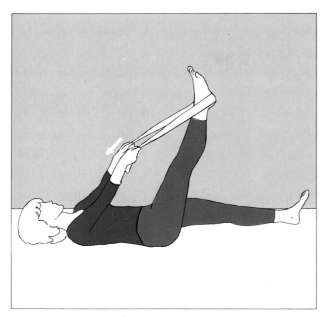

### 1 Stretching of the posterior thigh muscles

**Instructions**
- Wrap towel around heel
- With knee straight, bring leg up toward you as far as possible
- Against resistance, push leg in opposite direction with maximal contraction
- Bring leg further toward you

### 2 Stretching of the posterior thigh muscles and calf muscles

**Instructions**
- Wrap towel around the tip of the foot
- With knee extended, bring leg up toward you as far as possible
- Against resistance, push leg in opposite direction with maximal contraction
- Bring leg further toward you

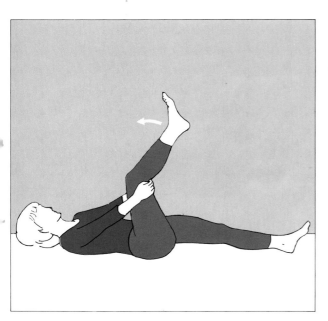

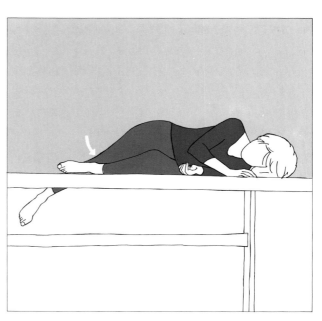

### 3 Stretching of the posterior thigh muscles

**Instructions**
- Bend leg at the knee and hold it in place with hands
- Straighten leg to a point where a pulling type of pain sensation is perceived in the posterior muscles
- Relax
- Repeat further straightening

### 4 Stretching of the lateral thigh muscle

**Instructions**
- With the leg closest to the table bent, lie on one side across the table at an angle
- Extend the other knee and drop that leg behind the posterior edge of the table
- Bring leg back up
- Relax and drop leg further

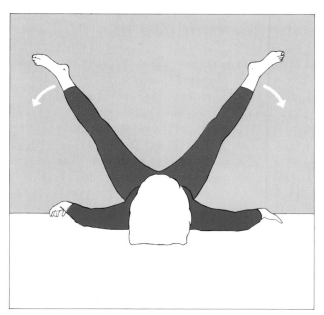

### 5 Stretching of the medial thigh muscles

**Instructions**
- Lie supine with buttocks and posterior thighs placed against the wall
- With knees straight, let legs move apart slowly
- Contract medial thigh muscles (as if wanting to bring legs together)
- Relax

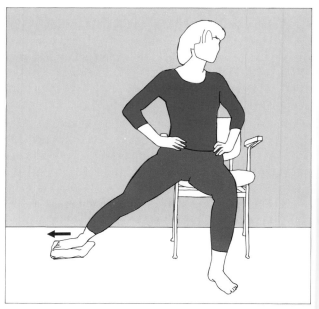

### 6 Stretching of the medial thigh muscles

**Instructions**
- With the knee straight, place one leg to the side, push medial foot margin against the floor
- Relax
- Allow leg to glide further outward

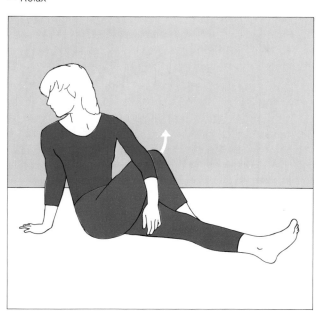

### 7 Stretching of the deep gluteal muscles

**Instructions**
- Pull knee toward opposite hip
- Against some resistance, push knee outward
- Relax
- Pull knee closer toward the opposite hip

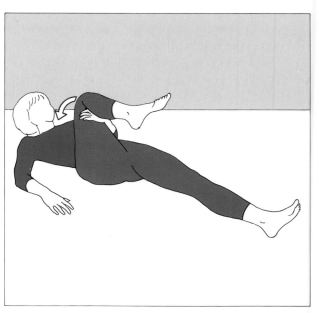

### 8 Stretching of the deep gluteal muscles

**Instructions**
- Pull knee with hand toward the opposite shoulder
- Against resistance, contract maximally as if wanting to move knee away from shoulder
- Relax
- Pull knee further toward the opposite shoulder

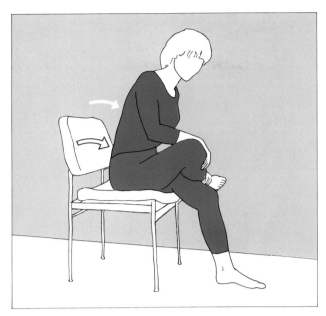

## 9 Stretching of the deep gluteal muscles

**Instructions**
- Pull knee toward opposite hip
- Straighten upper body while inhaling simultaneously
- While exhaling, lean forward with straight upper body
- Further straighten trunk, again while inhaling
- Repeat stretch

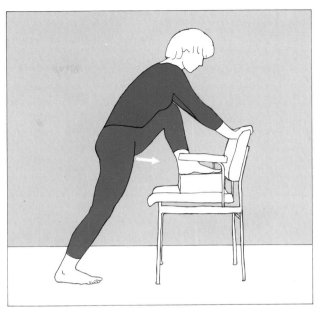

## 10 Stretching of the hip flexor muscles

**Instructions**
- Move pelvis forward over the extended support leg (the leg making contact with the floor)

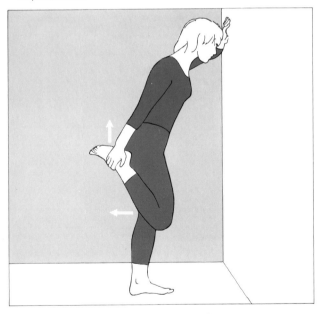

## 11 Stretching of the hip flexor and long knee extensor muscles

**Instructions**
- Pull leg up behind you
- Against resistance, straighten knee
- Relax
- Pull leg up further

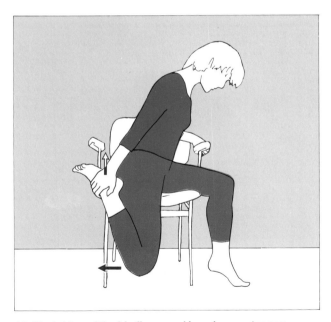

## 12 Stretching of the hip flexor and long knee extensor muscles

**Instructions**
- Pull leg up behind you
- Drop head forward
- Straighten knee against resistance
- Relax
- Pull leg up further

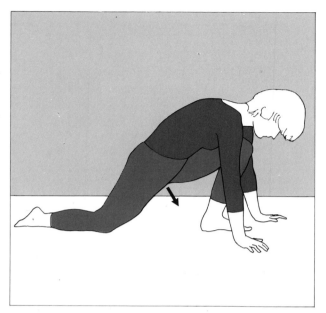

**13  Stetching of the hip flexor and long knee extensor muscles**

**Instructions**
- Assume position similar to that of starting for a sprint
- Push straightened (posterior) knee toward the floor
- Relax
- Extend hip further

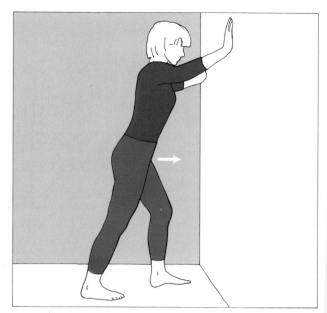

**14  Stretching of the calf muscles**

**Instructions**
- Lift heel of the posterior leg off the floor
- Push heel flat against the floor
- With the back straight, move trunk slowly forward
- Lift heel off the floor, then push it down again
- Stretch further

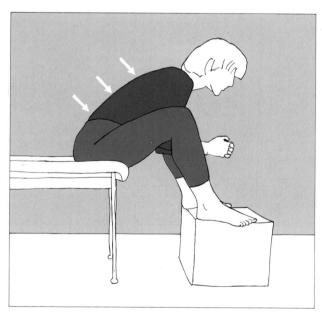

**15  Stretching of the lower back extensor muscles**

**Instructions**
- Sit with legs slightly apart and feet raised (i.e., on books, etc.)
- Lean upper body forward
- Inhale
- Exhale while pulling the arms below the chair
- Inhale and exhale
- Pull arms further below the chair

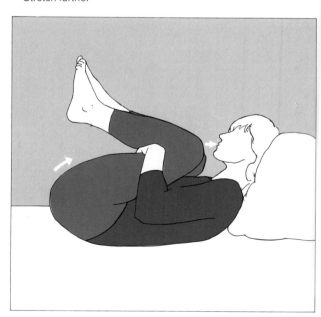

**16  Stretching of the lower back extensor muscles**

**Instructions**
- Bring knees toward the chin until the pelvis begins to lift off the floor
- Press thighs against arms and inhale
- Exhale and relax
- Bring knees further toward your chin

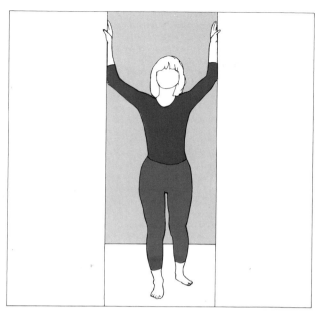

## 17  Stretching of the chest muscles

### Instructions
– Walking position
– Press hands against door frame
– Relax
– Lean upper body forward

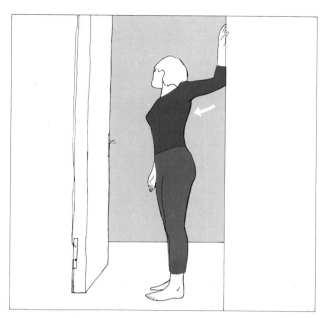

## 18  Unilateral stretching of the chest muscles

### Instructions
– Stand sideways to the door frame; rest forearm against the frame
– Press forearm against door frame
– Rotate trunk away (in small rotational steps) with the forearm remaining stationary

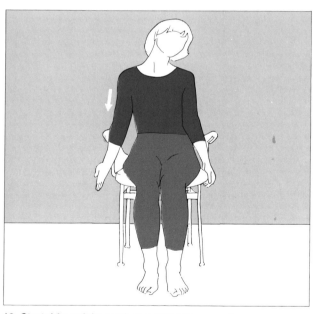

## 19  Stretching of the neck and shoulder muscles

### Instructions
– Bend head to one side
– Rotate arm outward and push it toward the floor
– Inhale and lift shoulder
– Exhale and pull arm toward the floor

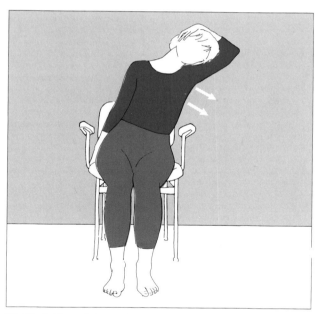

## 20  Stretching of the neck and shoulder muscles

### Instructions
– Bend head to one side (i.e., left) and hold in place with one hand
– Grasp chair with the other hand
– Lean trunk to the same side (i.e., left)
– Move back somewhat toward the original position and place hand on the chair closer to the floor
– Repeat side-bending of the trunk

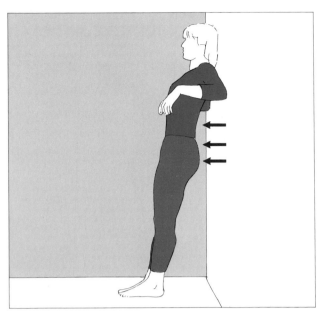

### 21 Strengthening of the shoulder blade muscles

**Instructions**
- Lean with shoulder blades against the wall at an angle
- Push trunk off with the elbows, while maintaining normal lumbar lordosis (do not arch back)

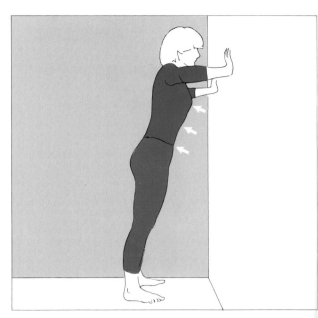

### 22 Strengthening of the shoulder blade muscles

**Instructions**
- Place fingertips against the wall at shoulder level
- Push body off slightly
- Maintain normal lumbar lordosis (do not arch back)

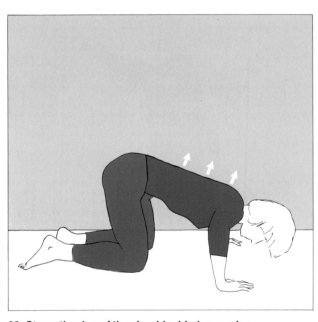

### 23 Strengthening of the shoulder blade muscles

**Instructions**
- Rest on knees and hands
- Slowly drop upper body between hands

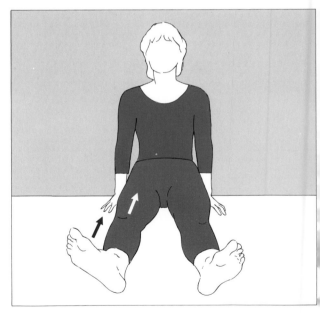

### 24 Strengthening of the anterior thigh muscles

**Instructions**
- Rotate leg slightly outward
- Keep knee straight
- Pull great toe and foot toward you
- Pull kneecap toward you
- Contract anterior thigh muscles

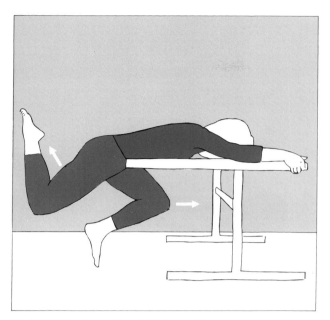

**25  Strengthening of the gluteal muscles**

**Instructions**
– Lift one leg (with knee bent) up toward the horizontal while
  pushing the opposite leg under the table top

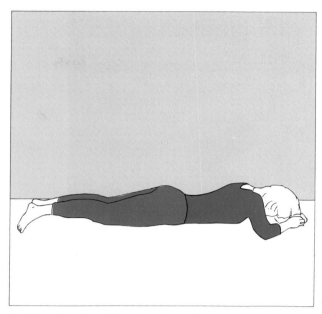

**26  Strengthening of the gluteal muscles**

**Instructions**
– Press heels together
– Contract buttock muscles maximally

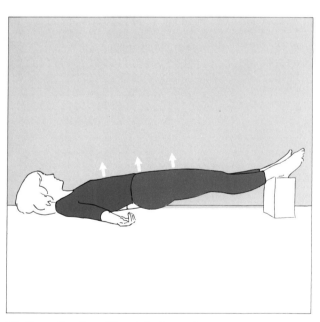

**27  Strengthening of the gluteal muscles**

**Instructions**
– Raise heels and rest them on support
– Contract buttock muscles and simultaneously lift pelvis and
  lower back off the floor

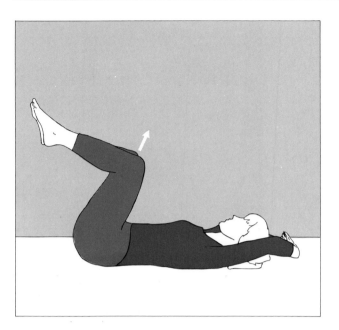

**28 Strengthening of the abdominal muscles**

**Instructions**
- Push knees toward the ceiling
- At the same time, lift pelvis slightly off the floor

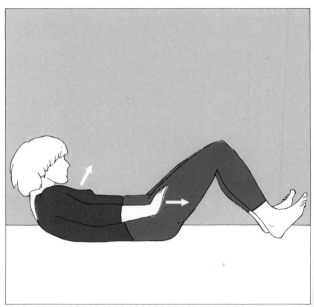

**29 Strengthening of the abdominal muscles**

**Instructions**
- Pull toes toward you while pressing heels against the floor
- Rotate arms slightly inward
- Bend hands upward and push in direction of the feet
- Lift head and shoulders off the floor

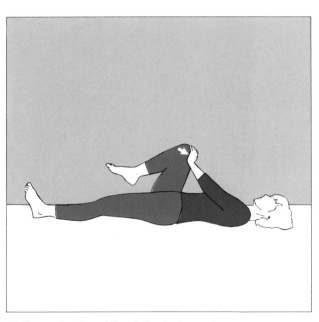

**30 Strengthening of the abdominal muscles**

**Instructions**
- Bend knee and press against resistant hand
- Slightly lift head off the floor

Translated by W.G. Gilliar, D.O. (with permission from F. Hoffmann-La Roche Company, Basel, Switzerland)

# Index

# Index